THE RUSH
INTERNAL MEDICINE
HANDBOOK

The Rush Internal Medicine Handbook

Editors
ROGER C. BONE, M.D.
KAREN A. GRIFFIN, M.D.

Associate Editor
KAREN B. WEINSTEIN, M.D.

Assistant Editors
KATHERINE MULLIGAN, M.D.
KEVIN CONLON, M.D.

From the Department of Internal Medicine,
Rush Medical College, Chicago, Illinois

YEAR BOOK MEDICAL PUBLISHERS, INC.
Chicago ● London ● Boca Raton ● Littleton, Mass.

3 4 5 6 7 8 9 0 R P 94 93 92

Library of Congress Cataloging-in-Publication Data

The Rush internal medicine handbook.

 Includes bibliographical references.
 1. Internal medicine—Handbooks, manuals, etc.
I. Bone, Roger C. II. Title: Internal medicine handbook.
[DNLM: 1. Internal Medicine—handbooks. WB 39 R952]
RC55.R87 1990   616   89-16730
ISBN 0-8151-1036-7

Sponsoring Editor: Richard H. Lampert
Assistant Director, Manuscript Services: Frances M. Perveiler
Production Project Coordinator: Karen Halm
Proofroom Supervisor: Barbara M. Kelly

The Editing Staff and Authors wish to dedicate this book to Dr. Stuart Levin. He has guided a generation of physicians through their residency training and taught them not only how to be academically astute physicians, but more importantly how to be good and caring doctors.

Contributors

Scott Adelman, M.D.

David Baldwin, Jr., M.D.

Jefferson Burroughs, M.D.

Herbert T. Cohen, M.D.

Larry Cripe, M.D.

Mark Dietz, M.D.

Jeffrey Dugas, M.D.

Ellen Glick, M.D.

William Hallmon, M.D.

Aaron Hamb, M.D.

Timothy Hines, M.D.

George Hvostik, M.D.

Mary Jacobs, M.D.

Rosemarie Jeffrey, M.D.

Nancy Lance, M.D.

James Lane, M.D.

Anthony Mannina, M.D.

Pat Murphy, M.D.

Susan Nadis, M.D.

Jeffrey Nelson, M.D.

Nina Paleologos, M.D.

Scott Palmer, M.D.

Stephen Paul, M.D.

Richard Petrak, M.D.

John Phelan, M.D.

Ed Priest, M.D.

Michael Rezak, M.D.

Sheldon Sloan, M.D.

R. Jeffrey Snell, M.D.

Peter Stein, M.D.

San San Wong, M.D.

Rebecca Wurtz, M.D.

From the Department of Internal Medicine, Rush Medical College, Chicago, Illinois

Preface

With the first edition of *The Rush Internal Medicine Handbook* we offer medical students and housestaff the opportunity to bridge the gap between the voluminous texts of internal medicine, and the bedside decision making of patient care. One of the most trying and important periods of our training is the transition from classroom to the medical ward. Unfortunately, experience in patient care cannot be obtained prior to medical clerkships and internships. The residents at Rush Presbyterian St. Luke's Medical Center (Chicago) put together this first edition in order to make easily available pertinent medical information to the student/physician in training.

Almost everyone who has undergone residency training in Medicine has kept notes, tables, algorithms and mnemonics in an attempt to remember the most relevant medical facts. This book represents a compilation of these facts. We have attempted to cover all the topics housestaff and students have considered most important in initiating and maintaining patient care, while keeping it in a pocketsize book.

It is with sincere gratitude to our authors that we offer this book to our readers.

Roger C. Bone, M.D.
Karen A. Griffin, M.D.

Acknowledgments

We wish to acknowledge the following persons for their contributions to this book:

John Principe, M.D./Pulmonary; Robert Balk, M.D./Infectious Diseases; Constance Benson, M.D./Nephrology; Roger Rodby, M.D./Gastroenterology; John Schaffner, M.D., Don Jensen, M.D./Allergy and Immunology; Allan Luskin, M.D., Wendell Richmond, M.D./Endocrinology; David Baldwin Jr., M.D./Formulary; Mary Ellen Carasiti, Pharm. D., Dwayne Keller, R.P.H., A. Rossof, M.D./Oncology; S. Rosenbush, M.D./Cardiology. We are also grateful for the expert secretarial assistance of Paula Brown and Lorraine Russell.

Roger C. Bone, M.D.
Karen A. Griffin, M.D.

Contents

14 **PROCEDURES** 343
Richard Petrak and Stephen Paul

Pulmonology

Richard Petrak, M.D.
Anthony Mannina, M.D.
Scott Palmer, M.D.

PULMONARY FUNCTION TESTS

Pulmonary function tests (PFT) can be helpful adjuncts to the clinical evaluation of patients. PFT are indicated in the following instances:

1. To establish baseline ventilatory function.
2. To follow the progression of a disease process.
3. To assist in the assessment of disease.
4. To monitor therapy.
5. Preoperatively in patients with known or suspected lung disease.
6. To determine the extent of impairment.
7. In patients at high risk of developing lung disease (e.g., smokers, occupational exposure, etc.).

The four general categories of assessment are spirometry, lung volumes, diffusion capacity, and arterial blood gases.

Spirometry measures forced expiratory volumes over certain periods of time (in other words, flow). With the nostrils closed, the patient is directed to take as deep a breath as possible and to blow into the spirometer as hard and fast as possible. Volume and time are measured on a kymograph from which various flows can be measured. The most common measurements are the following:

1. Forced vital capacity (FVC). This is the total amount of air expired during the forced expiratory maneuver described above.
2. Forced expiratory volume in 1 second (FEV_1). This is the amount of air expired during the first second of the spirogram.
3. Forced expiratory flow in the middle half of the spirogram (FEF_{25-75}). This is determined by measuring the flow rate of 50% of the FVC volume after 25% of the FVC has been expired. In other words, it measures the flow over the middle 50% of the FVC.
4. Maximal voluntary ventilation (MVV). This is the volume of air breathed over 12 seconds during which the patient breathes as deeply and rapidly as possible.

Restrictive lung diseases may cause a decrease in all spirometric measurements (Table 1-1). If restrictive lung disease is suggested or suspected, a determination of lung volume is indicated. Obstructive lung disease may also show decreases on spirometry. The sine qua non of obstructive lung disease is a decrease in the ratio of FEV_1 to FVC compared to normal. When findings of spirometry suggest obstructive lung disease, inhaled bronchodilators are administered and the forced expiratory maneuver is repeated. A response to bronchodilators is considered significant if spirography after bronchodilators shows an increase of 15% in either FEV_1 or FVC, or a 25% increase in FEF_{25-75}. MVV is decreased in people with neuromuscular disease or in those who make a poor effort.

Lung volumes are measured with helium dilution or body plethysmography. Body plethysmography should be performed when the findings of spirometry suggest the presence of obstructive lung disease. The most common lung volumes measured are the following:

1. Total lung capacity (TLC). This is the total amount of air present in the lungs after a maximal inspiration.
2. Functional residual capacity (FRC). This is the volume of air present in the lungs after a normal expiratory maneuver.

3. Residual volume (RV). This is the volume of air present in the lungs after a forced expiratory maneuver.

A decrease in TLC is the sine qua non of restrictive lung disease. TLC is normal or increased in obstructive lung disease. An increase in FRC suggests the presence of air trapping, while an increase in the ratio of RV to TLC with a decrease in MVV and no evidence of obstruction suggest neuromuscular disease or a poor effort by the patient.

The diffusion capacity of the lung for carbon monoxide (DL_{CO}) is a measure of the ability of the lungs to diffuse gas across the alveolar capillary membrane. DL_{CO} is decreased in emphysema, anemia, or when there is a decrease in lung volume.

DL_{CO} is increased in polycythemia, pulmonary hemorrhage, left-to-right cardiac shunts, and asthma. Arterial blood gases are discussed thoroughly in the section on acid-base balance.

ARTERIAL BLOOD GASES

1. Alveolar air equation:
$$PAO_2 = FI_{O2} (P_{ATM} - P_{H2O}) - (PaCO_2/0.8),$$
where
PAO_2 = partial pressure of O_2 in alveolar gas;
FI_{O2} = fraction of O_2 in inspired air;
P_{ATM} = atmospheric pressure = 760 mm Hg at sea level;
P_{H2O} = partial pressure of H_2O in inspired air;
$PaCO_2$ = partial pressure of CO_2 in arterial blood.
Alveolar to arterial (A-a) gradient = $PAO_2 - PaO_2$.

Estimated normal A-a gradient = $\dfrac{Age}{4} + 4$

PULMONARY THROMBOEMBOLISM (PTE)

Pulmonary thromboembolism is a complication of deep venous thrombosis (DVT). In 95% of cases, PTE arise from the deep

TABLE 1-1.
Diseases Causing Changes on Spirometry

Parameter	Causes of Decrease	Causes of Increase	Comments
Vital capacity	Restrictive lung disease	Obstructive lung disease	
FEV$_1$	Asthma, emphysema, chronic bronchitis	None	An improvement of ≥15% after a bronchodilator denotes a reversible component to obstructive lung disease.
FEV$_1$/FVC (%)	Asthma, emphysema, chronic bronchitis	Some restrictive lung disease	Eliminates restriction as a variable. Abnormal only in obstructive processes.
MMEF (FEF$_{25-75}$)	Chronic obstructive pulmonary disease, asthma	None	Measures disease in middle-sized airways.
MVV	Poor muscle function of chest wall or diaphragm, poor patient effort	None	Measures muscle endurance and ventilatory reserve.
Slow vital capacity	Emphysema, bronchospasm	None	A slow vital capacity ≥10% increase over FVC denotes air trapping.
FRC	Restrictive lung disease	Ankylosing spondylitis	Unaffected in neuromuscular disease.
RV	Space-occupying lesions, lung resection, restrictive lung disease	Expiratory muscle disease	Normal or increased in neuromuscular disease.

	Restrictive lung disease	Obstructive lung disease	Comments
TLC	Restrictive lung disease	Obstructive lung disease	Measures efficiency of ventilation.
RV/TLC	None	Neuromuscular or chest wall disease, poor patient effort	<80% of predictive value is abnormal.
DL_{CO}	Emphysema, interstitial lung disease, pulmonary vascular disease, resection of lung parenchyma, anemia	Congestive heart failure, polycythemia, intracardiac shunts, pulmonary hemorrhage, asthma	

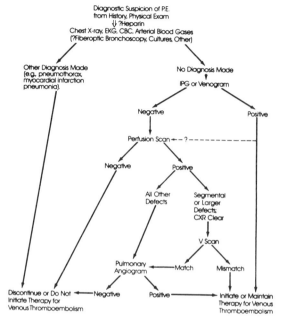

FIG 1-1
Diagnostic flowchart for PTE. (Adapted from Moser KM: Pulmonary thromboembolism, in Braundwald, Isselbacher, Petersdorf, et al (eds): *Harrison's Principles of Internal Medicine.* New York, McGraw-Hill Book Co, 1987. Used by permission.)

veins of the lower extremities (above the knee). Only 50% of patients with DVT have clinical signs or symptoms (Tables 1–2 and 1–3).

RISK FACTORS FOR DVT

Prolonged bed rest, carcinoma, obesity, estrogens, lower extremity fracture or other injury, congestive heart failure, postpartum period, chronic deep venous insufficiency, prior DVT or PTE, hypercoaguable states (e.g., antithrombin III deficiency, lupus anticoagulant, protein S and C deficiencies), advanced age, and nephrotic syndrome.

TABLE 1–2.
PTE

Symptoms	Incidence (%)	Signs	Incidence (%)*
Dyspnea	84	Tachypnea >20/min	85
Pleuritic chest pain	74	Tachycardia >100/min	58
Apprehension	63	Accentuated P$_2$	57
Hemoptysis	28	Rales	56
Syncope	4–17	Fever >37.5°C	50

*Based on 214 patients without prior cardiac or pulmonary disease in the Urokinase Streptokinase Pulmonary Embolism Trial (USPET).

TABLE 1–3.
Testing for PTE

Diagnostic Tests	Comments
DVT: Impedence plethysmography with Doppler studies	Highly sensitive above the knee; noninvasive
Radiofibrinogen scan	Highly sensitive below the knee
Contrast venography	Gold standard
PTE: Ventilation/perfusion (VQ) Scan	If perfusion scan is normal, PTE is excluded. High probability scan (multiple segmental or lobar defects with ventilation mismatch) has a 90% correlation with pulmonary arteriography

Findings on Tests

1. Arterial blood gases (ABG): shows $PaO_2 < 80$ mmHg in 90%; respiratory alkalosis is common.
2. Electrocardiogram (ECG): sinus tachycardia, T wave inversion, and nonspecific ST segment changes are most common; S_1Q_3, right axis deviation, right bundle branch block, and P pulmonale occur in less than 20%; and recent onset of atrial fibrillation occurs in less than 5%.
3. Chest x-ray (CXR): Findings are most commonly normal or may show an elevated hemidiaphragm, infiltrate, or oligemia on the side of the embolus (Westermarks sign); pleural based infiltrate (Hamptons hump) and a small pleural effusion may occur in pulmonary infarction.

These findings are most useful in ruling out other disorders rather than diagnosing PTE.

Since the therapy for PTE has significant risks involved with it, the diagnosis of PTE should be made as definitively as possible. The simplest examination to begin with is a nuclear medicine ventilation-perfusion scan. A normal perfusion scan rules out significant PTE. A high probability scan (i.e., one or more segmental or greater mismatched defects) will correlate positively with pulmonary angiography about 85% of the time. Pulmonary angiography remains the gold standard for demonstrating an intravascular thrombus but has definite risks involved with it. In a patient for whom the suspicion of PTE is high, the demonstration of DVT can lead one to make the presumptive diagnosis of PTE. The gold standard for diagnosing DVT is contrast angiography. A less invasive method is impedence plethysmography with Doppler (IPG/Doppler), which has a sensitivity of greater than 90% in demonstrating DVT above the knee. It is noteworthy that DVT is not found in the majority of cases with PTE.

I. Treatment
    A. Anticoagulation: Heparin initially (intravenous loading dose of 5,000 U followed by 1,000 U/hr to achieve a partial thrombophastin time (PTT) 1.5 to 2.0 times greater than the control for 7 to 10 days, after which warfarin may be used at a dosage to

achieve a prothrombin time (PT) 1.5 to 2.0 times
greater than the control. Warfarin should be started
early since it takes 3 to 5 days once PT is in the
therapeutic range to achieve an anticoagulant effect.
Follow up the PT initially every day until the desired level of anticoagulation is achieved.

B. Contraindications to anticoagulation include: Active
internal bleeding, recent cerebrovascular accident
(within 2 months), recent major surgery, recent obstetric delivery, recent gastrointestinal (GI) bleeding, recent serious trauma, and severe hypertension.

C. Thrombolytic therapy: Not shown to improve morbidity or mortality compared to anticoagulation.
May have a role in massive pulmonary embolism
with hypotension.

D. Vena cava interruption: Indications include massive
embolus when recurrence would be fatal, proven recurrent embolus after the first few days of anticoagulation therapy, and if heparin is absolutely
contraindicated. This procedure prevents future emboli, but does not promote resolution of existing
emboli.

PLEURAL EFFUSION

A posteroanterior chest radiograph may only show pleural fluid
if more than 300 mL is present. Removal of pleural fluid may
serve diagnostic and/or therapeutic purposes (Tables 1–4 and 1–
5). Diagnostic thoracentesis to remove a relatively small amount
of fluid should be performed when the cause of the effusion is
uncertain. Therapeutic thoracentesis, not to exceed 1,000 to 1,500
mL of pleural fluid, should be performed for relief of symptoms
or when known infection is present.

CHRONIC OBSTRUCTIVE PULMONARY DISEASE

Definitions

Emphysema.—(pathologic definition) disorder characterized

TABLE 1–4.
Diagnosis of Transudate vs. Exudate

Criteria	Transudate	Exudate
Lactic dehydrogenase (LDH): pleural fluid/serum	<0.6	>0.6
Protein level: pleural fluid/serum	<0.5	>0.5
Total LDH in pleural fluid	<200 U	>200 U
PH	>7.2	<6.8
Differential diagnoses	Congestive heart failure, nephrotic syndrome, hypothyroidism, constrictive pericarditis, cirrhosis with ascites, peritoneal dialysis	Infection, neoplasm, pulmonary embolism, pancreatitis, esophageal perforation, collagen vascular disease, Dressler syndrome, Meig syndrome, chylothorax

TABLE 1–5.
Studies Useful in the Diagnosis of Exudate

Study	Result	Comment
Cytologic studies	Malignant cells	Three separate fluid samples yield a diagnosis in 80%
	Mesothelial cells	Uncommon in tuberculosis (TB)
RBC	Grossly bloody (>5000 cells/mm³)	Pulmonary infarction, tumor, or trauma
Cell counts		
WBC	Neutrophil predominant	Acute inflammation: pneumonia, pancreatitis, pulmonary infarction, collagen vascular disease or subphrenic abscess
	Eosinophils >10%	Frequently due to air or blood in pleural space; occasionally due to parasitic or fungal infection; uncommon in TB
	Lymphocytes >50%	Malignancy or TB
Amylase level	>upper limit of normal for serum	Pancreatitis, esophageal rupture or malignancy
Glucose level	<60 mg/dL	TB, malignancy, rheumatoid disease, parapneumonic effusion, esophageal rupture
Triglyceride level	>110 mg/dL	Chylothorax, (+chylomicrons) or pseudochylothorax (–chylomicrons)
Chylomicrons		Chylothorax
Gram stain	Positive for organisms	Pleural space infection
Acid-fast bacilli smears	Positive	Positive in 20% to 30% of patients with TB pleurisy

TABLE 1–6.
Emphysema Versus Bronchitis

	Emphysema	Bronchitis
Etiology	Cigarette smoking, α-1 antitrypsin deficiency	Cigarette smoking (environmental and occupational exposure may play a minor role)
Symptoms	Progressive dyspnea	Cough and sputum production, episodic dyspnea
Physical examination	"Pink puffer", thin, no cyanosis	"Blue bloater", obese, may have cyanosis
Chest	↑ anteroposterior (AP) diameter and ↓ diaphragmatic excursion, ↓ breath sounds	AP diameter and diaphragmatic motion are normal, diffuse rales and rhonchi are present
Cardiac	Distant heart sounds	Heart sounds have normal intensity, may have an accentuated P_2 and signs of right ventricular failure
Chest X-ray	Hyperinflation, flattened diaphragm, ↑ retrosternal air space, bullous changes, small heart	Accentuated lung markings, cardiomegaly, ↑ pulmonary artery shadows
Laboratory	(−) erythrocytosis	(+) erythrocytosis
ECG	Low voltage	Right axis deviation, right ventricular hypertrophy, P-pulmonale
Arterial Blood Gases	$PaCO_2$ is normal, PaO_2 is decreased	$PaCO_2$ is increased, PaO_2 is decreased
Natural history	Progressive dyspnea, wasting, preservation of gas exchange; cor pulmonale and respiratory failure occur late	Relatively asymptomatic between exacerbations (usually due to respiratory tract infection), may have respiratory failure and right ventricular failure that reverse with treatment

by distention of the air spaces distal to the terminal bronchiole with destruction of alveolar septae.

Bronchitis.—(clinical definition) excessive mucus secretion manifested as a chronic or recurrent productive cough on most days for a minimum of 3 months a year for at least 2 consecutive years. The majority of patients will present with a mixture of emphysema and bronchitis and may have a component of asthma.

The two main objectives of therapy are to minimize or prevent intercurrent complications and to treat all reversible elements of the underlying disorder. Cessation of smoking is very important. Respiratory tract infections should be treated promptly. Beta-2 agonists inhaled anticholinergics and aminophylline should be used to control bronchospasm. Control of secretions can be attained with pharmacotherapy and physical therapy. Influenza and pneumococcal vaccines should be administered.

Severe hypoxia from a combination of hypoventilation and ventilation-perfusion mismatching requires oxygen therapy. PaO_2 should be maintained at greater than or equal to 55 to 60 mmHg with oxyhemoglobin saturation greater than 90%. It is essential to start with low flow oxygen so as not to depress ventilation further by withdrawing the hypoxic stimulus to breathe. Arterial blood gases must be monitored frequently. If acidemia and hypoventilation result from excess oxygen, supplementary oxygen should be decreased but not discontinued.

ASTHMA

Asthma is an episodic and largely reversible disease characterized by tracheal and bronchial hyperactivity associated with reversible mucosal edema. The pathophysiologic changes may reverse spontaneously or with therapy. Asthmatic patients may be divided into two clinical groups, intrinsic and extrinsic, with extrinsic accounting for less than 10% of patients. More than 80% of asthmatics have characteristics common to both clinical groups.

I. Clinical manifestations
    A. History: Elicit history of atopy, age of onset, frequency and duration of attacks, medication compliance, provocative stimuli*, steroid dependence,

---

*Provocative stimuli include respiratory tract infections (viral bronchitis, only rarely pneumonia), air pollutants, occupational inhalants, exercise, cold air, emotional factors, aspirin or non-steroidal anti-inflammatory drugs. Sampter syndrome is the triad of bronchospasm, nasal polyps, and aspirin sensitivity.

TABLE 1–7.
Classification of Asthma

Extrinsic	Intrinsic
Known external allergens	No known external allergens
Positive skin tests	Negative skin tests
Elevated IgE levels	IgE not elevated
Onset in children/young adults	Onset in adults (usually >35 years old)
Attacks are acute, and may be severe but are easier to control	Attacks are fulminant, and difficult to control
History of childhood eczema	No childhood eczema
Family history of asthma	No family history of asthma
Peripheral eosinophilia	Aspirin sensitivity
	Peripheral eosinophilia

      prior hospitalizations, emergency room visits, and prior intubation.

  B. Physical examination: Examine for tachycardia, tachypnea, diaphoresis, restlessness, wheezing, use of accessory muscles of respiration, and a pulsus paradox greater than 18 mmHg. The latter two findings correspond to severe disease, corresponding to an FEV_1 of less than 25%. NOTE: absence of wheezing (a silent chest) is an ominous sign.

II. Laboratory evaluation

  A. Sputum: Wet prep for eosinophils and Charcot-Leyden crystals.

  B. Arterial blood gas:

Severity of attack	pH	PCO_2	PO_2
Mild	↑	↓	Normal or ↓
Moderate	Normal	Normal or ↓	↓
Severe	↓	↑	↓ ↓

  C. ECG: May show P-pulmonale, right ventricular hypertrophy, right bundle branch block, right axis deviation.

    D. Chest x-ray: Assess for hyperinflation, atelectasis secondary to mucous plugs, infiltrates, pneumothorax, or pneumomediastinum.

    E. Pulmonary function tests: Measurement of FEV_1 and peak expiratory flow rate provide objective evidence as to the severity of the attack and response to therapy.

III. Differential diagnosis: Includes congestive heart failure, chronic bronchitis, pulmonary embolus, large airway obstruction, and laryngeal edema.

IV. Therapy: For mild attacks, inhaled β-2 agonists are generally effective. Theophylline may be given at relatively low doses, as there is an additive effect when a β-2 adrenergic agent is combined with theophylline. If there is little response or the attack becomes more severe, hospitalization is indicated for intravenous theophylline and steroids (solumedrol, 125 mg or hydrocortisone, 200 mg every 6 hours), as well as inhaled bronchodilators. When the patient has responded clinically to therapy, medications can be converted to oral preparations, such as prednisone 60 mg per day. Steroids can be tapered over 2 to 3 weeks.

ADULT RESPIRATORY DISTRESS SYNDROME
Definition

ARDS (adult respiratory distress syndrome) is a common clinico-pathophysiologic disorder that is characterized by:

1. The abrupt onset of marked dyspnea.
2. Progressive hypoxia.
3. Decreasing lung compliance.
4. Evolution of bilateral pulmonary infiltrates on chest x-ray.

Etiology

ARDS is seen following a wide variety of noxious insults to the pulmonary parenchyma and can also occur after seemingly unrelated events in the body. Through a sequence of common pathophysiologic events, these insults then mediate the development of increased pulmonary capillary permeability and subsequent accumulation of extravascular fluid (water and plasma proteins). ARDS affects an estimated 150,000 people per year in the United States and the mortality rate, despite the latest therapeutic interventions, remains greater than 60%.

Causes of ARDS include:

1. Shock states (septic*, cardiogenic).
2. Infection (bacterial, viral, fungal, protozoal, mycobacterial).
3. Drug or toxin exposure (including smoke inhalation and oxygen toxicity).
4. Trauma (burns, fractures, head injury, lung contusion).
5. Aspiration (gastric acid, near-drowning).
6. Miscellaneous (leukoagglutinin reaction, eclampsia, high altitude, pancreatitis).

Clinical Presentation

ARDS should be suspected following the recognition of these signs and symptoms:

1. Sudden onset of pronounced dyspnea and tachypnea (especially after possible inciting event).
2. Intercostal retractions with use of accessory muscles.
3. Hypoxia refractory to oxygen therapy (suggestive of shunt physiology: decreased PaO_2 on an $FIO_2 \geq 40\%$).
4. Development of diffuse patchy infiltrates on early chest x-rays with evolvement into a dense bilaterial interstitial and/or alveolar pattern within 24 to 72 hours.

ARDS is a syndrome in which the diagnosis depends on both the fulfillment of the above criteria plus the exclusion of: left ventricular failure (grossly defined as pulmonary wedge pressure > 18 mmHg); diffuse pulmonary infection; and advanced chronic obstructive pulmonary disease.

---

*Most common overall cause of ARDS.

Treatment

The management of ARDS is mainly supportive in nature; that is, attempting to maintain adequate tissue oxygen delivery by providing respiratory and circulatory support, while treating the underlying disease. The therapeutic goal is to maintain this support until the integrity of the alveolar-capillary membrane can be reestablished. However, the prevalence of multi-organ failure and recurrent sepsis in these patients contributes greatly to the overall mortality of ARDS despite optimal care. The essential tenets of care include:

I. Maintain adequate tissue oxygenation: Although many different clinical parameters are useful to monitor patients, the one which seems the best is the calculation of arterial oxygen transport:

$$\text{Arterial oxygen transport} = \text{cardiac output} \times \text{arterial oxygen content}$$

Optimization of arterial oxygen transport through the above relationship calls into consideration a number of variables that may be quickly modified in an acute setting. Arterial oxygen content is calculated as:

$$(PaO_2 \times 0.03) + (\text{Hemoglobin} \times 1.34 \times \text{Arterial } O_2 \text{ saturation})$$

From the above equation, the intrinsic importance of measuring serial arterial blood gases (or at least arterial oxygen saturations) can be seen. The importance of measuring the hemoglobin level can also be seen (must be > 10g), since the right side of the above equation contributes most of the total arterial oxygen content. Positive end-expiratory pressure (PEEP) is very helpful in the setting of ARDS. It seems to increase arterial PO_2 levels and allows a reduction of the FIO_2. The physiologic consequences of PEEP are:

1. Prevention of distal airway closure on expiration, thus increasing pulmonary compliance and the functional residual capacity.
2. Oxygenation of previously closed airways by alveolar recruitment with optimization of ventilation/perfusion mismatching in these alveolar units.
3. Reduction in cardiac output via increased intrathoracic pressures and decreased cardiac preload.

This last physiologic effect, via the arterial oxygen transport equation, may result in a net reduction in overall oxygen delivery to the tissues. It may be partially overcome, however, with the infusion of fluids and use of inotropic agents. It is therefore useful, when changing PEEP settings with ARDS, to always calculate the effect of such changes on arterial oxygen transport.

Other useful clinical parameters to assess when treating patients with ARDS are: mixed venous oxygen tension and the difference between arterial and venous oxygen content; and pulmonary compliance.

II. Optimize pulmonary wedge and arterial pressures:
Through the use of Swan-Ganz catheterization, measurements of these values (including cardiac output) can be easily performed and monitored to minimize the accumulation of interstitial fluid while maintaining adequate tissue perfusion. Note that the use of PEEP in this setting may falsely elevate recorded wedge readings, and should be discontinued for recordings only.

III. Treat underlying causes (if possible): Potentially treatable causes of ARDS include pulmonary or other infections, vasculitic disorders, metabolic derangements and immunologically-mediated diseases. The prophylactic use of antibiotics is not indicated in most cases.

IV. Experimental/controversial treatments:
   A. Prostaglandin inhibitors: known to mediate the inflammatory response of a variety of stimuli. Early studies have shown that meclofenamate and ibuprofen can prevent an increase in airway resistance and a decrease in dynamic pulmonary compliance after

the experimental infusion of endotoxin.

B. E-series prostaglandins: PGE$_1$ and PGE$_2$ have been shown to decrease lymphokine production, induce T-lymphocyte suppressor activity, and diminish macrophage toxic oxygen radical production. Recent trials with PGE$_1$ in patients with ARDS have reportedly resulted in improved survival rates.

C. Corticosteroids: previous data have shown that steroids will inhibit platelet aggregation and release of arachadonic acid byproducts in sheep infused with endotoxin. However, recent multicenter clinical trials have failed to demonstrate any beneficial effects of methylprednisolone on the reversal of diagnostic criteria for sepsis-induced ARDS or on survival rates.

ACUTE RESPIRATORY FAILURE

Acute respiratory failure (ARF) occurs when the pulmonary system is unable to meet metabolic demands. The patient is usually acutely dyspneic and may exhibit disorientation, lethargy, or coma. The diagnosis however often rests on arterial blood gas analysis, which shows PaO$_2$ <50 mmHg, PaCO$_2$ >50, and pH <7.30.

The treatment of ARF consists of establishment of an airway, administration of oxygen (Tables 1–9, 1–10), and maintenance of adequate ventilation. Then one can identify and treat the underlying condition, while monitoring patient's progress.

The main indications for mechanical ventilation are ventilatory failure as indicated by a rising PaCO$_2$ and/or severe hypoxemia that cannot be corrected with high concentrations of inspired oxygen.

Mechanical ventilation: The ventilator mode must be chosen according to which of three breathing modes is desired. Settings are approximate and should be adjusted based on arterial blood gases and the clinical setting (Table 1–11). The three modes are: Assist/control ventilation, in which a predetermined minimum respiratory rate is set, and the patient may initiate additional breaths, each of which triggers a fixed volume ventilator breath; intermittent mandatory ventilation (IMV), in which a predetermined ventilator breath rate is set in between which the patient is allowed

TABLE 1-8.
Differential Diagnosis of ARF

Type	Mechanism	Site of Involvement	Example
Hypercapnic-hypoxemic with Normal A-a gradient	Hypoventilation due to respiratory center depression	CNS	Sedative drug overdose, cerebral vascular accident, cerebral trauma, CNS tumor
	Hypoventilation due to insufficient chest wall function	Spinal cord	Spinal cord trauma, Guillian-Barré, poliomyelitis, amyotrophic lateral sclerosis, myasthenia gravis, muscular dystrophy, tetanus or botulism, hypokalemia, hypophosphatemia, hypomagnesemia, kyphoscoliosis, trauma with flail chest, obesity
	Hypoventilation due to upper airway obstruction	Upper airway	Epiglottitis, laryngeal edema, tracheal obstruction

Hypercapnic-hypoxemic with increased A-a gradient	Inability to excrete CO_2 due to VQ mismatch	Lung parenchyma and airway	Chronic bronchitis, emphysema, asthma
Hypoxemia with hypocapnea	VQ mismatch and shunt	Lung parenchyma	ARDS, congestive heart failure, overwhelming pneumonia

TABLE 1–9.
Oxygen Delivery Systems*

Method of Administration	FIO$_2$
Nasal canula (1–2 L)	.24–.28 (approximate)
Venturi mask	.24, .28, .35, .40, .50
Partial rebreathing reservoir mask	.60–.80
Nonrebreathing reservoir mask	Up to .90
Endotracheal tube	Any concentration up to 1.0

TABLE 1–10.
Guidelines for Ventilatory Support in ARF*

Data	Normal	Intubation and ventiliation indicated
Respiratory Rate (resp/min)	12–20	>35
Vital capacity (mL/kg)	65–75	<15
FEV$_1$ (mL/kg)	50–60	<10
Max inspiratory force (cm H$_2$O)	75–100	<25
PaO$_2$ (mmHg)	75–100	<60 with FIO$_2$>.6
PaCO$_2$ (mmHg)	35–45	>55 (unless chronic)

The trend of values is important and numerical guidelines should never replace clinical judgment.
*From Pontoppidan et al: *Acute Respiratory Failure in the Adult. N Engl J Med* 1972.

to take normal spontaneous breaths; and controlled ventilation, in which the ventilator delivers a preset respiratory rate regardless of patient effort.

Weaning From Mechanical Ventilation

Weaning should be considered after the respiratory emergency is stabilized. Weaning should not be attempted until arterial blood gases are stable, fluid and electrolyte balance is normal, and infections are controlled (Table 1–12). No one technique of weaning (T tube versus IMV) has clearly documented superiority. Weaning is likely to be successful if the following criteria are met: vital capacity $\geq$ 10–15 mL/kg; tidal volume $\geq$ 5–10 mL/kg; resting minute ventilation $\leq$ 10 L/minute; negative inspiratory pressure at least -20 cm H_2O; and maximum voluntary ventilation more than twice minute ventilation.

TABLE 1–11.
Ventilator Settings

Setting	Description
Tidal volume	Usually 10–15 mL/kg
Respiratory rate (RR)	8–15/min (to keep $CO_2 = 40$) Adjustment can be made with: Desired RR = Previous rate × Previous PCO_2/Desired PCO_2
FIO_2	Lowest amount required to maintain PaO_2 = 60.
Positive end expiratory pressure (PEEP)	Increases end expiratory lung volume (FRC) and reduces shunting in ARDS. Maintain at lowest level necessary to keep $paO_2 >$ 60 with $FIO_2 < .60$.

Pressure Measurements

Plateau pressure (PP)	Measured during a brief inspiratory hold. At a given tidal volume, it reflects the compliance of the chest wall and lung parenchyma. Increased plateau pressure may indicate pulmonary edema, pneumonia, pneumothorax, or right mainstem intubation.
Peak pressure	Reflects properties of the entire system (lung, chest wall, and airways). Increasing difference between plateau and peak pressures reflects increased airway resistance (eg, bronchospasm, mucus plug, endotracheal tube blockage, etc.).

TABLE 1–12.
Complications in Patients Requiring Mechanical Ventilation

Complication	Prevention and/or Therapy
Right mainstem intubation	Deflate cuff and pull back
Esophageal intubation	Deflate cuff, extubate, and re-intubate
Tracheal stricture	Perform tracheostomy after 14–21 days of tracheal intubation
Pneumothorax	Chest tube placement; decrease PEEP
Pneumomediastinum	Decrease PEEP
Subcutaneous emphysema	Decrease PEEP
Decreased cardiac output	Decrease PEEP
Rapid acid-base shifts	See renal section
Oxygen toxicity	Keep $FIO_2 < 60\%$
Upper GI bleeding	See GI section

SARCOIDOSIS

Definition

A multisystem granulomatous disorder of unknown etiology characterized by the presence of noncaseating granulomas.

Clinical Features

Sarcoidosis occurs mostly in young adults, with a ratio of women to men of 2:1 and a black-to-white ratio of 10:1. Organ involvement in declining order of frequency are lungs, mediastinal lymph nodes, peripheral lymph nodes, skin, eyes, and liver. However, any organ system can be involved.

Usual types of presentation:

1. Asymptomatic: 30% to 40% of cases are discovered with a routine chest x-ray.
2. Respiratory: manifested by cough, dyspnea, hemoptysis, fever, and malaise.
3. Löefgren's syndrome: abnormal chest x-ray (hilar adenopathy) associated with a triad of erythema nodosum, large-joint polyarthralgias, and uveitis. It is an acute, self-limiting variant mediated by high levels of circulating immune complexes.

Diagnosis

A diagnosis is attained by recognizing the constellation of presenting signs and symptoms in association with the presence of noncaseating granulomas on a biopsy specimen (taken from peripheral lymph nodes, lung tissue, skin lesions, or liver tissue). Other granulomatous disorders, however, should be excluded (e.g., tuberculosis, fungal disease, berylliosis).

Chest X-ray Findings

Stage	Findings on CXR	Found at presentation (%)	Remission (%)
0	Normal	5–16	
I	Bilateral adenopathy	25–40	60
II	Bilateral adenopathy with infiltrates	24–49	40
III	Infiltrates without adenopathy	6–15	12
IV	Parenchymal fibrosis	uncommon	rare

Laboratory Findings

A. Kveim test: an intradermal injection of tissue derived from known sarcoidosis victims. An area of induration connotes a reaction to the Kveim-Siltzbach antigen and is confirmed by the observation of typical granulomas on a biopsy specimen.
Disadvantages of the test are the overall unavailability of the antigen, the need for a biopsy after 4 to 6 weeks and its relatively low sensitivity with regard to chronic sarcoidosis.

B. Angiotensin converting enzyme (ACE) assay: levels are elevated due to a byproduct of epitheloid cells in sarcoid granulomas. Correlates more with the presence of granulomas rather than with active inflammation.
Specificity limited by false-positive results seen with miliary TB, leprosy, Gaucher's disease, and hyperthyroidism.

C. Gallium scan: ^{67}Ga uptake by activated pulmonary macrophages correlates with the intensity of alveolitis. False-positive results are seen with interstitial pneumonia, silicosis, and asbestosis.
D. Other lab findings:
   1. Hypercalcemia and hypercalciuria (slightly more common).
   2. Hyperglobulinemia.
   3. Hyperuricemia.
   4. Abnormal pulmonary function tests (restrictive lung disease).
   5. Elevated erythrocyte sedimentation rate, Raji cell and Clq binding assays (secondary to increased circulating immune complexes).
   6. Positive rheumatoid factor.
   7. Increased viral titers.
   8. Cutaneous anergy.
   9. Abnormal liver function tests.
   10. Conduction abnormalities on ECG.

Treatment

Sarcoidosis is generally a benign, self-limited disease requiring no specific treatment. However, the following medications may be efficacious:

A. Prednisone (1 mg/kg for at least 4 to 6 months). Indications include:
   1. Ocular involvement.
   2. Myocardial involvement with conduction disturbances.
   3. Central nervous system involvement.
   4. Severe respiratory disease.
   5. Disfiguring cutaneous lesions.
   6. Persistent elevation of serum and/or urine calcium; seen in about 10% of patients.

   Consider the concurrent use of isoniazid if patient is anergic or PPD positive.
B. Chloroquine (500 mg/day). Indications include:
   1. Hypercalcemia.
   2. Cutaneous lesions.

   Mechanism of action is inhibition of 1α-hydroxylase produced by the granulomas.

Infectious Diseases 2

Jeffrey Nelson, M.D.
Ellen Glick, M.D.
Timothy Hines, M.D.
Rebecca Wurtz, M.D.

INFECTIVE ENDOCARDITIS

Classification

The terms acute and subacute were used in the past to define the various clinical presentations seen with this disease. Acute referred to disease caused by more virulent organisms such as *Staphylococcus aureus*, often involved normal valves, and had a more fulminant clinical course. Subacute generally referred to infections with the *Streptococcus* viridans group of organisms from the mouth, involved previously damaged valves, and had favorable clinical outcomes. More recently, these terms have been replaced with a more precise classification of patients based on the organism involved and the host. These two features help define therapy and prognosis with greater clarity.

History

1. Recent dental work may provide a clue for a viridans streptococcal organism.
2. A carbuncle or other staphlococcal skin infection may be a clue to *S. aureus*.
3. Genitourinary or gastrointestinal instrumentation may precede enterococcal endocarditis.
4. Endocarditis occurring after recent prosthetic valve surgery may be due to coagulase-negative staphylococci, enterococci, or gram-negative bacilli.

5. Patients with liver disease are at greater risk for endocarditis due to gram-negative organisms.
6. Intravenous drug usage increases the likelihood of staphylococci, gram-negative bacilli, and fungal organisms.

Physical Examination

1. Petechiae on conjunctivae, palate, and lower extremities.
2. Painful Osler's nodes representing emboli on digits.
3. Macular erythematous Janeway lesions on palms and soles.
4. Hemorrhages with central pallor (Roth spots) on funduscopic examination.
5. Splinter hemorrhages on nails.
6. Palpable spleen.
7. Fever and a murmur are usually present.

Laboratory

1. Elevated sedimentation rate and anemia are the most common findings.
2. Urinary findings of hematuria or proteinuria occur in 50% of patients.
3. Elevated white count can be seen but need not be present.
4. Rheumatoid factor and circulating immune complexes can be seen in more chronic forms.

Diagnosis

1. Three blood cultures obtained over several hours will demonstrate more than 95% of bacteremias associated with endocarditis. With three positive results, one must consider the presence of persistent bacteremia of an endothelial origin. In most patients, this implies endocarditis.
2. An echocardiogram is quite specific if one sees a vegetation, but less than 50% sensitive for endocarditis.
3. Occasionally, one may look for evidence of embolization as an indirect clue to the diagnosis of endocarditis. A liver-spleen scan may be helpful.

Pathogens

1. Viridans streptococci from the mouth are perhaps the most common isolates.
2. *S. aureus* is also quite common and it is often associated with intravenous drug usage.
3. Enterococci account for less than 20% of isolates. They are associated with genitourinary manipulation.
4. Gram-negative pathogens are increasingly more common in intravenous drug abusers and hospitalized patients.
5. Fungal endocarditis is seen primarily in intravenous drug users and patients with prosthetic valves.

Culture Negative Endocarditis

Occasionally the clinical presentation suggests endocarditis but no pathogen is isolated. The most common cause is previous antibiotic therapy. Others include: fastidious organisms, fungal disease, and rarer causes such as *Chlamydia*.

Treatment

1. *S. aureus*:
   a. Oxacillin or nafcillin if community acquired. A possible exception is the intravenous drug user in whom methicillin-resistant *S. aureus* is becoming increasingly common.
   b. Vancomycin if it is a hospital-acquired organism or if the patient is allergic to penicillin.
   c. Four to six weeks of intravenous treatment is recommended.
2. Viridans streptococci: Penicillin G, 10–12 million units per day, for 4 weeks of intravenous treatment. This may be shortened to 2 weeks if an aminoglycoside is used with the penicillin.
3. Enterococci: No single drug is adequate. Recommended therapy requires two drugs, usually ampicillin and gentamicin. Vancomycin can be substituted for ampicillin in the penicillin-allergic patient. Treatment is for 6 weeks.
4. Gram-negative organisms: A single drug may be adequate but with *Pseudomonas*, double coverage is optimal. An aminoglycoside or a third generation

cephalosporin is often used. Treatment is for 4 to 6 weeks.

5. Fungal: Amphotericin B is the recommended therapy. The duration of therapy is dose related and dependent on the type of fungus. Surgery is often as needed.

Surgical Intervention

While all pathogens have the potential to lead to valvular failure, there are those which more commonly require surgery for cure. These include those with fungal and gram-negative organisms as pathogens and patients with prosthetic valves. Indications for surgery include: persistent bacteremia, systemic emboli, and congestive heart failure. Since an individual's disease progression is often unpredictable, cardiothoracic surgical consultation is often warranted.

PNEUMONIAS

Etiology

The common community acquired bacterial pathogens to be considered are the following: *Streptococcus pneumoniae*, *Hemophilus influenzae*, *Legionella*, *S. aureus*, and *Mycoplasma pneumoniae*. In the debilitated host (alcoholic, elderly, chronic obstructive pulmonary disease), the following organisms should also be considered: (1) Oropharyngeal anaerobes: *Fusobacterium*, *Peptostreptococcus*, *Peptococcus*, *Bacteroides*; (2) Gram-negative rods: *Escherichia coli*, *Klebsiella*, *Enterobacter*, *Pseudomonas*, *Serratia*; (3) *Staphylococcus*.

The patient with neutropenia is prone to a myriad of pathogens, but gram-negative rods are prime suspects. In the acquired immune deficiency syndrome, *Pneumocystis carinii* is a first consideration when interstitial pneumonitis is present.

The acquisition of pneumonia in the hospital setting prompts consideration of other likely organisms: *S. aureus*, gram-negative rods, and *Legionella*.

Diagnosis

I. Sputum:

A. Gram's stain: A good specimen has less than 10 ep-

  ithelial cells and greater than 25 white cells per
  100 × field. If a predominant organism is seen, it
  offers another clue to the diagnosis.

 B. Culture: Only useful if it is from an adequate sputum sample confirmed with Gram's stain to minimize contamination by oral flora.

 C. DFA: Direct fluorescent antibody test uses antibody
  to detect *Legionella* antigens. It is a very specific
  test, but is only about 30% sensitive.

 D. CIE: Counterimmunoelectrophoresis helps detect antigens of *S. pneumoniae* and *H. influenzae* with a
  gel diffusion method. Results are available in hours
  and are very specific, but again are only about 30%
  sensitive.

 E. AFB: Smear and culture if TB is suspected.

 II. Blood cultures: At least two should be obtained. While
 not very sensitive, a positive culture result is quite specific.

 III. Pleural fluid: Very specific and, if occurring with *Staphylococcus* or gram-negative organisms, is fairly sensitive.

 IV. Serology:

 A. CIE: As with sputum, one can find antigens in sera.

 B. IFA: Immunofluorescent antibody test is used to detect antibody titers to *Legionella*, a titer of 1:124 or
  a fourfold rise in convalescent titer is considered
  positive.

 C. Cold agglutinins: IGM antibody to the I antigen on
  RBC is seen in 50% of cases with mycoplasma.

Treatment

With the above information, one can sometimes strongly suspect
a single pathogen. The following are examples of possible intravenous antimicrobial regimens:

1. Pneumococcus: Procaine penicillin G, erythromycin.
2. *Legionella*: Erythromycin or doxycycline.
3. *H. influenzae*: Ceftriaxone or ampicillin (20% are resistant to ampicillin).

4. Staphylococcus: Oxacillin or vancomycin.
5. Anaerobes: Clindamycin or penicillin.
6. Gram-negative organisms: Aminoglycoside or ceftazidime.
7. Pneumocystis: Sulfamethoxasole and trimethoprim, or pentamidine.

Often no specific pathogen can be decided on to guide initial treatment. Empiric treatment must then be started. Possibilities include the following:

1. Community acquired pneumonia in a normal host: Erythromycin.
2. Community acquired pneumonia in a debilitated host: Add cefotaxime to erythromycin.
3. Nursing home or recently hospitalized host: Add ceftazidime to erythromycin.
4. Neutropenic host: Amikacin and ceftazidime.
5. Acquired immune deficiency: Trimethoprim sulfamethoxazole.

Initial treatment can be changed as laboratory data suggest a specific cause. Should the patient not respond to initial treatment, more invasive diagnostic procedures may be necessary with a reevaluation of initial therapy.

OSTEOMYELITIS

Symptoms
Localized pain may be the only symptom. In acute osteomyelitis, one may see systemic symptoms of fever and toxicity.

Risk Factors
Trauma, surgery, joint prostheses, drug abuse, overlying soft tissue infection, sickle cell disease, diabetes, and chronic vascular insufficiency.

Diagnosis
1. Acute osteomyelitis may be associated with bacteremia. Isolation of an organism precludes the need for a bone

biopsy. Frequently acute osteomyelitis does not have an associated bacteremia, therefore, these cases, as well as chronic osteomyelitis cases, necessitate a bone biopsy to isolate the pathogen.

2. An x-ray of a bone may show characteristic bone changes to suggest osteomyelitis. These changes require more than a week before they are evident.

3. A bone scan will often show uptake in the first few days and is, therefore, a more sensitive test early in the infectious course.

Organisms

S. aureus is the most common isolate. *Staphylococcus epidermidis* occurs frequently in the postoperative orthopedic patient. Sickle cell disease predisposes the patient to salmonella infection particularly of the vertebrae. Diabetics and those with vascular insufficiency are prone to mixed infections including anaerobes and gram-negatives organisms. Spinal disease is often due to tuberculosis.

Treatment

Acute osteomyelitis generally requires about 4 to 6 weeks of intravenous antimicrobial therapy. Chronic disease requires a more prolonged course of 8 to 12 weeks and often several months. Empiric therapy for acute osteomyelitis usually requires agents active against *S. aureus*. Those with diabetes or vascular insufficiency should also be given therapy for gram-negative and anaerobic organisms. Timentin or clindamycin and an aminoglycoside are possible treatments when mixed infections occur. Treatment can be simplified once the pathogen and its sensitivities are known.

URINARY TRACT INFECTIONS

Asymptomatic Bacteriuria

This infection occurs in 2% to 5% of women in the child-bearing years, 2% to 10% of women who are pregnant, and in 5% to 15% of older women. No specific organism is causative. Treatment is necessary if the woman is pregnant, has diabetes, or a predisposition to renal disease (eg, polycystic kidney).

Acute Uncomplicated Cystitis

This infection occurs in healthy young women. There is an absence of fever, flank pain, and systemic symptoms. Causative organisms include: *E. coli* and *Staphylococcus saprophyticus*. Single-dose therapy or a 7-day course of oral antibiotics is necessary.

Relapsing Urinary Tract Infections

This occurs when the same organism reinfects the patient. No specific organism is causative. Radiologic and urologic evaluation is necessary. In men, prostatitis should be considered and treated for 6 to 12 weeks.

Reinfection

This occurs when different organisms reinfect the patient. If this occurs infrequently, it should be treated as a single infection with a single dose of short-term therapy. If it occurs frequently, 6 months to 2 years of prophylactic therapy should be administered.

Complicated Infections

This occurs with kidney stones, urologic manipulation, and with an indwelling catheter. With kidney stones, the causative organisms are: *Proteus*, *Klebsiella*, and enterococci. With manipulation or an indwelling catheter, causative organisms include *Proteus*, *Klebsiella*, *Pseudomonas*, *Serratia*, enterococci, and fungi.

Laboratory Evaluation

I. Microscopic examination of urine:
   More than five to 10 white blood cells per high-power field in centrifuged sediment.
   More than 20 bacteria per high-power field in centrifuged sediment.
   More than one bacterium per high-power field in uncentrifuged urine.
   WBC casts usually indicate an upper urinary tract infection (UTI).

II. Urine culture:
   Mandatory in evaluation of upper UTI. Usually more

than 100,000 bacteria per mL, but may be symptomatic
with less than 100,000 bacteria per mL. Must culture
after therapy to document success of treatment.

III. Blood cultures:
Mandatory in upper UTI. If cultures remain positive,
consider obstruction or perinephric abscess.

IV. Intravenous pyelography indications:
Any child with first UTI.
Adult man with first UTI.
Adult woman with frequent UTI.
Nonresponsive pyelonephritis.

Empiric Therapy

The ultimate therapy depends on the results of urine culture.

I. Lower UTI.
  A. Conventional treatment: 7 to 10 days with ampicil-
     lin, cephalexin, or trimethoprim-sulfamethoxasole.
  B. Single-dose treatment: amoxicillin 3.0 g orally or
     trimethoprim-sulfamethoxasole double strength once
     orally.

II. Dysuria without bacteriuria (consider *Chlamydia* or *Neis-
seria gonorrhea).
Tetracycline for 7 days.

III. Acute pyelonephritis.
If severely ill, parenteral cephalosporin plus parenteral
aminoglycoside. If less severely ill, parenteral cephalosporin alone or parenteral ampicillin or trimethoprim-sul-
famethoxasole.

IV. Prophylaxis.
Nitrofurantoin 50 mg or one-tab single strength trimetho-
prim-sulfamethoxasole or norfloxacin 400 mg daily.

DIARRHEA

Diarrheal illnesses can be generally divided into two major groups,
inflammatory and noninflammatory (Table 2–1). Inflammatory
causes usually produce colonic involvement, are invasive, and
are characterized by the presence of white blood cells in the stool.

TABLE 2–1.
Common Causes of Infectious Diarrhea

Organism	Risk Groups	History	Stool	Incubation	Treatment
Campylobacter	Travelers	Abdominal pain prominent	+ WBC, often blood	3 d, course: 3 d–2 wks	If severely ill, erythromycin
Shigella	2-3 yr olds	Elevated temperature prominent	Generally more blood	24 to 72 hr, course: last up to 2 wk	TMP-SMX*
Salmonella	2-3 mo olds, food borne outbreaks	Cramping, abdominal pain	(+) WBC, often blood	8-48 hr, course: 2–4 wk	Ampicillin if severe
E. coli Invasive		Bloody stool	Occult blood (+) WBC	12-72 hr	TMP-SMX*
Toxin mediated			Watery (−) WBC		
C. difficile	Travelers	Fevers, abdominal pain, history of antibiotic use	(+) WBC usually	Often prolonged with treatment	Oral/intravenous metronidazole or oral vancomycin
Norwalk (virus)	Less than 3 yr old	Watery stool	(−) WBC	Self limited	Rehydration
Rotavirus (virus)	6-18 mo olds	Watery stool	(−) WBC, + rotazyme	Self limited	Rehydration
Giardia (flagellate)	Untreated water	Less than 1 week bloating, flatulence	−WBC	Often asymtomatic	Metronidazole

| Cryptosporidium (protozoan) | Young children in day care, AIDS | Acute outbreaks, chronic in homosexuals | Special isolation | Chronic in AIDS, benign and self limited in normal host | Spiramycin (experimental), no effective therapy |

*TMP-SMX: trimethoprim-sulfamethoxazole.

Infections not explained by above causes:
A. Persistent pain/fever: Yersinia culture with cold enrichment.
B. Chronic bloody diarrhea: amoeba versus Giardia.
C. Seafood exposure: Special vibrio culture with cold enrichment.
D. Homosexual: Chlamydia, syphillis, gonorrhea, herpes.

Noninflammatory diseases generally involve small bowel, are noninvasive, and produce a watery stool without WBC. Below are some of the common pathogens in each group:

1. *Inflammatory*: *Campylobacter, Shigella, Salmonella, Clostridium difficile, Entamoeba histolytica,* invasive *E. coli* (uncommon), *Yersinia.*
2. *Noninflammatory*: Rotavirus, Norwalk virus, *Giardia, S. aureus,* toxigenic *E. coli, Vibrio cholera,* (non-cholera vibrios) *Clostridium perfringens,* and *B. cereus.*

The noninflammatory disorders, with the exception of *Giardia lamblia,* tend to be self limited and therefore require no specific workup or treatment. When seeing a patient with diarrhea, clues to prompt further evaluation should include the presence of WBC in the stool, fevers and abdominal pain, duration of symptoms greater than 1 week, and recent ingestion of antibiotics.

Initial workup should include a stool sample for methylene blue staining to look for WBC and a stool sample for ova and parasites. Stool cultures are reserved for those in the inflammatory group (ie, WBC in stool).

Treatment in general is primarily fluid replacement. Specific treatment is sometimes needed in severe cases.

In a severely ill patient with an inflammatory diarrhea, a reasonable antimicrobial regime might include bactrim or erythromycin.

In a patient with a history of previous antibiotic therapy, stool should be assayed for *C. difficile* toxin. If positive, treatment with oral flagyl or vancomycin should be initiated.

FEVER OF UNKNOWN ORIGIN

Definitions

Fever of greater than 3 weeks' duration, with a temperature greater than 101°F, and no proven etiology after 1 week of workup.*

Etioiogies

A few general categories constitute most etiologies:

*Adopted from Beeson, Petersdorf *Medicine* 1961.

1. Tumors: hematologic most common.
2. Infectious: abdominal abscesses, TB, and HIV infection are important.
3. Connective tissue diseases.
4. Granulomatous diseases.
5. Drugs.

*Workup

The most important part of the workup is repeated history and physical examinations focusing further tests on one's findings. Other helpful simple tests include:

1. Complete blood count: looking for evidence of lymphoma, leukemia, and infection.
2. Urinalysis: Hematuria and pyuria may be helpful clues.
3. Erythrocyte sedimentation rate: significant elevations over 100 make tumor, connective tissue disease, or chronic infection likely.
4. Three sets of blood cultures to help rule out endocarditis.
5. Tuberculosis skin test.
6. Chest x-ray.
7. Gallium scan.

Further Course

Screening tests often guide you to further testing, which may include a bone marrow examination, computed tomography of the abdomen, liver biopsy, skin and muscle biopsy, and sinus radiographs.

Some fevers remain undiagnosed and if suspicion is high for a particular process, therapeutic trials of antibiotics, non-steroidals, anti-tuberculous drugs, or steroids may be necessary.

NEUTROPENIA

Definition

Profound granulocytopenia is defined as the presence of less than 500 granulocytes, calculated as white blood cells × percentage of polymorphonuclear cells and bands.

Etiology

Includes acute leukemia, bone marrow transplantation, use of immunosuppressive drugs, and aplastic anemia.

The risk of infection increases with the duration of neutropenia. There are several other factors that combine with neutropenia to predispose the patient to infections: mucosal damage from chemotherapy, skin trauma (venipuncture, Hickman catheter, etc), and tumor obstruction.

The most common sites of infection in the neutropenic are the oropharynx, skin, lung, and perianal area. The organisms are those that usually colonize the infected area. Bacteremia without an obvious source is also common. The infection may be community acquired or nosocomially acquired (patient hospitalized within last 3 weeks).

A. Bacteria
  1. *Staphylococcus* species (most common isolate).
  2. Enteric gram-negative bacilli (formerly most common isolates).
  3. Anaerobes (very uncommon).
  4. TB and atypical mycobacteria.

B. Fungi
   Candida, Aspergillus, Mucor, Cryptococcus species.

C. Intracellular organisms
   Listeria and salmonella.

Workup

Workup includes routine cultures and sensitivity testing for positive cultures, chest x-ray, inspection of the rectal area, good skin and mucosa examination with attention to icthyma gangrenosum associated with *Pseudomonas* or other gram-negative bacilli, herpes vesicles, and periodontal disease. Check the retina for findings consistent with fungal disease and Roth spots. Further workup may include bronchoscopy if lung infiltrates are present, and endoscopy if the patient has esophagitis.

Empiric Treatment

Broad spectrum antibiotics:* Aminoglycoside plus an extended

---

*The key to initial therapy and good clinical outcome has been two drug gram negative coverage.

spectrum penicillin or third generation cephalosporin with anti-pseudomonas activity. Consider vancomycin for methicillin-resistant staphylococci. If there is no response after 48 to 72 hours, add amphotericin.

ACQUIRED IMMUNE DEFICIENCY SYNDROME (AIDS)

Definition and Description

AIDS is characterized by immune abnormalities, opportunistic infections, and unusual tumors. The causative agent is a retrovirus, human immunodeficiency virus (HIV) with HIV-1 being most commonly isolated from infected patients. The primary underlying defect is viral damage to the T4 helper cells. Because of this cell's central role in both cellular and humoral immune function, a number of immunologic abnormalities result.

Risk groups were originally confined to homosexuals, Haitians, intravenous drug abusers, and blood recipients. More recently, this risk group has been expanded to include the heterosexual contacts of individuals in high-risk groups, infants of HIV seropositive mothers, and health care workers.

Because of this increasing epidemic, there are certain precautions health care workers should observe. These have been updated in the Morbidity-Mortality Weekly Report (MMWR), August 21, 1987. While the virus can be isolated from numerous body fluids, only blood, semen, and vaginal secretions have been implicated in transmission thus far. Most important for prevention of disease transmission is to assume that all patients are potentially infected. The precautions one must take primarily involve barrier protection.

Gloves are important when working with open wounds, mucosal surfaces, bodily excretions, and blood products. Specific circumstances may make eyewear, gowns, or masks appropriate.

The definition of AIDS is under constant revision. The most recent Centers for Disease Control (Atlanta) update is found in the MMWR August 14, 1987 issue. HIV antibody status, specific unusual infections and neoplasms, and absence of other known immunodeficiency states all play a role in the diagnosis.

While HIV itself can cause specific disease syndromes such as encephalopathy, dementia, and a wasting syndrome, most pa-

TABLE 2–2.
Most Common Pathogens in AIDS Opportunistic Infections

Pathogen	Presentation	Diagnosis	Treatment
Pulmonary			
P. carinii	Insidious onset of shortness of breath, hypoxia, and fever. Chest x-ray may be clear or show diffuse infiltrates	Silver stain of sputum, bronchoalveolar lavage	TMP-SMX or Pentamidine
Cytomegalovirus	Similar to pneumocystis	Biopsy showing cellular inclusions	Ganciclovir 9(1-3 dihydroxy-propoxymethyl guanine)
Mycobacterium avium intracellulare	Similar to pneumocystis. Usually disseminated organ system disease with GI tract disease or involvement as common manifestations	Positive acid-fast smear and culture	Based on in vitro susceptibilities (no proven therapy-experimental regimen)
Central Nervous System			
Human immunodeficiency virus	Progressive encephalopathy	Cerebrospinal fluid (CSF) culture for HIV, elimination of other causes	Zidovudine
JC papovavirus	Progressive encephalopathy	Computed tomography (CT) scan with multiple hypodense white matter lesions, biopsy	No proven therapy

Cryptococcus neoformans	Headache; can present as meningitis, rarely focal deficits	India ink of CSF, cryptococcal antigen, and culture of CSF	Amphotericin B
Toxoplasma gondii	Often focal deficits	CT demonstrates multiple enhancing lesions; magnetic resonance imaging may be more sensitive; biopsy	Pyrimethamine plus sulfadiazine; folinic acid additionally
Gastrointestinal			
Candida	Oral ulcerations, esophageal complaints, odynophagia	Culture oral lesions, endoscopy and culture to rule out herpes which can present similarly	Clotrimazole; if esophageal, use amphotericin or ketoconazole
Cryptosporidium	Prolonged diarrhea	Modified acid-fast stain of stool for cryptosporidium	No therapy
Cytomegalovirus	Bloody diarrhea	Colonoscopy and biopsy of punctate ulcers showing inclusions	Ganciclovir
Ocular			
Cytomegalovirus	Visual complaints	Ophthalmologic examination	Ganciclovir
T. gondii	Visual complaints	Ophthalmologic examination	Pyrimethamine with a sulfadiazine

tients are hospitalized because of opportunistic disease (Table 2–2). The more common infectious presentations involve the lungs, central nervous system, eyes, and the GI tract.

TUBERCULOSIS (TB)

Conditions

1. Favoring primary pulmonary TB: renal dialysis, transplantation, crowded living conditions, alcoholism, pulmonary silicosis, and nursing home patients.
2. Favoring extrapulmonary TB: alcoholism, cirrhosis, HIV infection, and neoplasm. Most patients with miliary TB have no prior history of TB.
3. Favoring reactivation: gastrectomy, steroid therapy, HIV infection, and chemotherapy.

Diagnosis

1. History of exposure, cough, hemoptysis, weight loss, sweats, and fevers.
2. Chest x-ray: early apical patchy infiltrate, later apical cavitation, advanced widespread cavitation, infiltrates, and pleural effusion.
3. Culture/acid-fast bacilli (AFB) stain: sputum (early morning, obtain 3 to 5 specimens), urine, gastric aspirate (early morning), bronchoscopic specimen, bone marrow biopsy, pleural biopsy, and CSF if indicated.
4. PPD: intracutaneous injection of 0.1 mL of 5TU PPD (must raise a wheal). Should place in conjunction with an anergy profile. The test is read 48 to 72 hours later. A positive test is >10 mm induration. If the TB test is negative or equivocal and TB is still suspected, the PPD should be repeated with 250TU PPD.

Respiratory Precautions

Patients with AFB-positive sputum are contagious, but prolonged exposure and close contact are necessary for transmission to occur. It is sufficient to ask the patient to cough into a tissue and keep his door closed. In most cases, masks are not necessary. Linen and waste paper precautions are not necessary.

Therapy

Standard regimen for pulmonary TB includes: isoniazid (INH) 300 mg every day plus rifampin (RMP) 600 mg every day for 18 to 24 months. Streptomycin 1 g every day can be added for patients with extensive pulmonary involvement and should be continued for 2 months or until sputum is proven with an AFB smear to be free of the bacilli.

I. Short course (becoming standard)
   A. INH 300 mg plus RMP 600 mg every day for 9 months
      Optional: Ethambutol (EMB) 15–18 mg/kg or streptomycin (STM) 1 gm every day until sensitivity is known (especially in patients who have history of prior treatment, cases acquired in southeast Asia, Central America or Africa, and contact with a case known to have a resistant organism).
   B. Studies show that if INH and RMP are given daily for 2 months and the patient is AFB smear negative, the remaining 7 months of therapy can be given on a twice weekly basis with RMP 600 mg plus INH 900 mg.

II. Miliary TB: INH and RMP plus EMB or pyrazinamide (PZA) if, on epidemiologic grounds, the chance of resistant organisms is high: pending culture sensitivity results.

III. Pregnant women: INH, EMB for 18 to 24 months. Add RMP in advanced disease. Avoid STM (ototoxic).
   When is the Patient no Longer Contagious? Probably within the first 2 weeks of therapy. Optimally, when the acid-fast bacillus smear or culture is negative.
   Follow-up Studies
   A. Ideal: check sputum AFB smear after 1 month and every 2 weeks until conversion occurs.
   B. Practical: check sputum every 2 months until conversion occurs.
   C. Check liver function tests every 2 months for patients on INH (increased risk of hepatotoxicity in daily drinkers, patients on RMP, and those older than 35 years).

D. Follow up visual acuity in patients on ethambutol and perform audiography in patients taking streptomycin. After therapy is finished, some experts suggest a total of 2 years' observation with a chest x-ray and sputum AFB stain every 3 to 6 months.
Prophylactic regimen
The following should receive prophylaxis with INH for 1 year:

A. Household contacts with 5 mm skin test and no previous history of reaction. Household contacts who are children, especially those under 5 years of age, should be treated for 3 months even if the skin test is negative. At 3 months, repeat the skin test and if it is negative, treatment may be discontinued.
B. Newly infected patients or those with skin test conversion from negative to positive in the past 2 years.
C. Past history of tuberculosis, now inactive, not previously treated with adequate chemotherapy.
D. Positive skin test and abnormal chest x-ray, some data suggest these patients have low-grade disease and should receive two-drug combination therapy.
E. Positive skin test and the presence of silicosis, diabetes, prolonged corticosteroid treatment or other immune suppression, Hodgkin's disease, AIDS, and end-stage renal disease.
F. Positive skin test under 35 years of age.

BIBLIOGRAPHY

Aids

Grant IH, Armstrong D: Management of infectious complications in acquired immunodeficiency syndrome. *Am J Med* 1986; 81:59–72.
Morbidity and Mortality Weekly Report. August 14, 1987; 36:1–15.

Morbidity and Mortality Weekly Report. August 21, 1987; 36:1–18.

Diarrhea

Blackow NR, Cukor G: Viral gastroenteritis. *N Engl J Med* 1981; 304:397–406.
Guerrant RL, et al: Evaluation and diagnosis of acute diarrhea. *Am J Med* 1985; 78:91–98.

Endocarditis

Kaye D: Prophalaxis for infective endocarditis: An update. *Ann Int Med* 1986; 104:419–423.
King K, Harkneis JL: Infective endocarditis in the 1980s. *Med J Aust* 1986; 144:536–540, 588–594.

Fever of Unknown Origin

Larson EB, et al: Fever of undetermined origin: diagnosis and follow-up of 105 cases, 1970-1980. *Medicine* 1982; 61:269–292.

Meningitis

Benson, et al: Acute neurologic infections. *Med Clin North Am* 1985; 69:399–413.

Neutropenic Host

Schimpff SC: Overview of empiric antibody therapy for the febrile neutropenic patient. *Rev Infect Dis* 1985; 734–739.

Osteomyelitis

Wald ER: Risk factors for osteomyelitis: The past decade. *N Engl J Med* 1980; 303:360–370.

Pneumonia

McKellar P: Treatment of community acquired pneumonias. *Am J Med* 1985; 79:25–31.

Tuberculosis

Am Rev Resp Dis 1981; 123:343–358.
Stead WW: Present chemotherapy of tuberculosis. *J Infect Dis* 1982; 146:698–704.

Nephrology

Herbert T. Cohen, M.D.
Jefferson Burroughs, M.D.
George Hvostik, M.D.

RENAL DISEASE

Acute Renal Failure

Definitions

Acute renal failure - a clinical syndrome of progressive azotemia, occurring over hours to several days, and sometimes accompanied by a decreased urine output.

Anuria - less than 150 ml urine/24 hours

Oliguria - less than 450 ml/24 hours, or less than 150 ml/8 hours

General Concepts

Often, acute renal failure occurs in an easily recognizable clinical setting following an acute precipitating event, as listed in Table 3–1; however, acute renal failure may be more insidious in onset and multifactorial, particularly with prolonged hospitalization in a critical care setting. Management consists of early recognition and correction of unfavorable influences on the kidney, a search for an etiology (particularly treatable causes) with anticipation and treatment of the metabolic consequences of diminished renal function:

 I. Initial management:
    A. *First* send urine for electrolytes before administering diuretics or fluid replacement. Premature therapy without baseline urine chemistries can obscure very important information (see below).

B. Rule out obstructive uropathy; catheterize bladder, ultrasound abdomen.

C. Establish euvolemia (avoid overhydration).

D. Discontinue potentially nephrotoxic agents.

E. Treat severe hypertension

F. Attempt to reestablish urine flow.

    1. Fluid bolus 200 to 300 cc of 0.9% sodium chloride (NaCl) over 20 to 30 minutes (only if the patient is dehydrated).

    2. Trial of diuresis in incremental doses of diuretic at 20 to 30 minute intervals: 40, 80, then 160 mg of furosemide by intravenous push (IVP); 50 mg of ethacrynic acid, then 100 mg by IVP, and if necessary, the addition of 5 to 10 mg of metolazone orally.

    3. Renal perfusion doses of dopamine (2–5 mcg/kg/minute)

G. Consider specific treatment, i.e., alkalinize urine in setting of rhabdomyolysis or acute uric acid nephropathy.

II. Determination of etiology

A. Review the history, physical examination, laboratory data, medications, and recent tests and procedures.

B. Review the peripheral smear for evidence of hemolysis, suggestive of a microangiopathic process.

C. Consider local and systemic diseases.

D. Determine chronicity of renal failure.

    1. Normal hemoglobin suggests new onset renal failure.

    2. Small echogenic kidneys on ultrasound suggest chronic renal disease.

E. Examine urine for evidence of active sediment or infection.

    1. Red blood cell (RBC) casts suggest glomerular damage.

    2. White blood cell (WBC) and epithelial casts suggest renal interstitial damage.

F. In the oliguric setting, distinguish prerenal azotemia

from renal failure by comparing urine and serum chemistries (note: these indices only determine if the renal response is appropriate and should not substitute for a thorough physical exam:*)

	Uosm	UNa	UCr/PCr	FENa†
Prerenal	>500	<20	>40	<1
Renal	<350	>40	<20	>1

$$^\dagger FENa = \frac{UNa}{PNa} \div \frac{UCr}{PCr} \times 100.$$

   G. Workup for specific etiologies includes:
   1. Serum eosinophilia for acute interstitial nephritis or atheroembolic disease
   2. Urine dipstick for blood in the absence of RBCs, serum creatine phosphokinase (CPK), and urine myoglobin for rhabdomyolysis
   3. Antinuclear antibody (ANA), complement, and anti-DNA antibody for systemic lupus erythematosus
   4. Antistreptolysin O (ASO) titer, complement, anti-DNase B, and antihyaluronidase for poststreptococcal glomerulonephritis (acute and convalescent titers)
   5. Urine immunoelectrophoresis for detection of light chains in multiple myeloma
   6. Consideration of renal biopsy for cases of glomerulonephropathies.

III. Further management: anticipation and treatment of the metabolic consequences of renal failure
   A. Review medications and change dosage of or discontinue renally cleared drugs.
   B. Provide adequate nutrition (see nutrition section).

*UOsm = urinary osmolality; UNa = urinary sodium; UCr = urinary creatinine; PCr = plasma creatinine; FENa = fractional excretion of sodium; PNa = plasma sodium.

TABLE 3–1.
Common Causes of Acute Renal Failure

	Features
Contrast-induced	Occurs within 24 hr of exposure, usually nonoliguric; can have FENa <1; risk factors include renal insufficiency, diabetes, dehydration, and multiple myeloma
Aminoglycosides	Occurs during the second week of therapy, is usually nonoliguric, and is insidious in onset
Nonsteroidal anti-inflammatory drugs	Has renal hemodynamic effect in patients with preexisting renal disease or dehydration; also causes syndromes of hyperkalemia, interstitial nephritis, and proteinuria
Acute interstitial nephritis	Often includes a clinical syndrome of rash and fever with eosinophilia and eosinophiluria; is common with sulfas, β-lactams, allopurinol, and phenytoin
Acute tubular necrosis	Occurs in clinical settings of hypotension, surgery with anesthesia, sepsis, and hemorrhage; FENa >1
Obstructive uropathy	Occurs in association with prostatic hypertrophy, intra-abdominal tumors, nephrolithiasis, and retroperitoneal fibrosis; often is anuric but can be polyuric if partial, can have FENa <1
Acute GN	Often includes a clinical syndrome of edema, tea-colored urine, and hypertension with azotemia, proteinuria, and RBC casts in urine; can have FENa <1
Tumor lysis syndrome	Occurs with necrosis of a large tumor burden, as in leukemias and lymphomas, often related to initiation of chemotherapy; is usually oliguric
Hepatorenal syndrome	Occurs in the presence of severe hepatic insufficiency; usually is oliguric, with UNa <5; is diagnosis of exclusion

   C. Follow weights, fluid intake, and output.

   D. If patient is oliguric, replace fluids 1 cc per 1 cc plus insensible losses (100–200 cc) every 8 hours. Do not replace fluids if the patient is volume-overloaded.

   E. Limit intake of K^+, Na^+, and protein (if non-nephrotic) (see nutrition section).

   F. Keep serum bicarbonate greater than 10 mEq/L.

   G. Follow values of electrolyte, blood urea nitrogen (BUN), creatinine, blood pH, calcium, phosphorus, and magnesium.

   H. Consider dialysis for intractable:

     1. Acidosis

     2. Hyperkalemia (see fluid and electrolyte section)

     3. Volume overload

     4. Symptoms of uremia

     5. Toxic drug levels

   I. Watch for evidence of gastrointestinal (GI) bleeding, infection, and pericarditis.

Hematuria

Definitions

Men - greater than three RBCs/high-power field (hpf)
Women - greater than four RBCs/hpf

General Concepts

Normally, 1,000 RBCs/minute are lost in the urinary tract. A loss of 3,000 RBCs/minute is two standard deviations above the norm and results in the above criteria for significant hematuria; hence, these values are important clues for the presence of urinary tract pathology. Blood loss can occur anywhere along the urinary tract from the glomerulus to the urethral meatus. The goal of evaluation is to rule out the presence of significant disease, usually urologic but sometimes renal, specifically cancer (Table 3–2).

Proteinuria

Definitions

Significant proteinuria - greater than 150 mg/24 hours
Nephrotic-range proteinuria - 3.0 gm or more/24 hours

TABLE 3–2.
Etiologies of Hematuria Based on Clinical Setting and Urinary Features

Clinical and Urinary Features	Site	Etiologies*
Edema, hypertension, with proteinuria and RBC casts	Glomerulus	Glomerulonephritis (GN)
Flank pain, hematuria	Kidney or high urinary tract	Stones, renal vein thrombosis, renal infarction, papillary necrosis, tumor, and acute GN
Isolated hematuria	Kidney or urinary tract	Tumor, sickle cell anemia, hereditary nephritis, IgA nephropathy, benign prostatic hypertrophy and essential hematuria
Hematuria with clots	Urinary tract	Trauma, instrumentation, tumor
Hematuria with pyuria	Urinary tract > kidney	Pyelonephritis, cystitis, prostatis, urethritis

*Each of the etiologies listed may be present in more than one clinical setting.

Significant proteinuria (semiquantitative) - 2 + or 100 mg/dl or more by dipstick

General Concepts

Proteinuria is often a clue for the presence of renal disease, its mechanisms are outlined in Table 3–3. The extent to which evaluation and treatment are necessary varies with the clinical setting in which it occurs and the degree of proteinuria.

Large amounts of proteinuria often result in systemic metabolic complications (nephrotic syndrome), requiring full evaluation and often renal biopsy, as do the clinical syndromes of progressive renal failure with proteinuria and systemic inflammatory illness with proteinuria. These three clinical syndromes are associated with mild to severely aggressive glomerular disease and may require specific therapies. Lesser amounts of proteinuria (< 2 gm/24 hours) in the absence of these syndromes, considered isolated proteinurias, are generally tubular in origin.

Approach to the Patient

I. Initial evaluation
   A. Repeat dipstick (urinalysis)
   B. If 2 + or more proteinuria:
      1. Check 24-hour urine sample for protein value and creatinine clearance (if serum BUN and creatinine values are stable).
      2. Check serum creatinine, BUN, electrolytes, glucose, albumin, and cholesterol values.
      3. Check 24-hour urine immunoelectrophoresis for light chains.
      4. Check urine culture.

II. Subsequent evaluation: If syndromes of nephrotic-range proteinuria, renal insufficiency with proteinuria, or systemic inflammatory illness with proteinuria are present, extensive workup is necessary to look for secondary and treatable causes of renal disease.
   A. Antinuclear antibody, complement, and anti-DNA antibody for lupus nephritis.
   B. Antistreptolysin O titer, complement, anti-DNase B, and antihyaluronidase for poststreptococcal glomerulonephritis.
   C. Do workup for chronic infection: hepatitis B, osteomyelitis, endocarditis, intra-abdominal abscess.

TABLE 3–3.
Mechanisms of Proteinuria

Site	Mechanism	Etiologies*
Systemic disease	Overproduction of a filtered protein	Light chains of multiple myeloma, lysozyme in leukemia
Renal disease	Hemodynamic	
	Increased filtration of protein associated with decreased renal plasma flow	Congestive heart failure and diabetes mellitus
	Glomerular	
	Increased permeability of glomerular capillary wall, often due to immune complex disease	Glomerulonephritis, nephrotic syndrome
	Tubular	
	Decreased reabsorption of normally filtered proteins	Interstitial nephritis, heavy metal toxicity
Postrenal disease	Bleeding or exudation of plasma proteins from the collecting system	Severe urinary tract infection

*Lists of etiologies are not all inclusive.

  D. Do age-appropriate screen for occult malignancy.
  E. Consider fat aspirate and Congo red stain for amyloid.
  F. Evaluate for evidence of diabetes and hyperlipidemia.

Nephrotic Syndrome (NS)

The NS consists of a triad of findings: edema, proteinuria (>3.0 gm/24 hours), and hypoalbuminemia; its most common causes are listed in Table 3–4. The NS implies the presence of a glomerular lesion that alters its ability to exclude protein from the urine while allowing a relatively preserved glomerular filtration rate (GFR).

In adults, primary, or "idiopathic," NS accounts for two thirds of cases and secondary diseases for one third. Primary causes are listed by renal biopsy morphology. Similar glomerular lesions can be seen in secondary disease as well, as in membranous nephropathy due to chronic hepatitis B antigenemia or with penicillamine therapy.

Complications that may result from a loss of immunoglobulin, antithrombin III, and vitamin D carrier protein in the urine include, respectively, infection, renal vein thrombosis, pulmonary embolism, and hypovitaminosis D. The hyperlipidemia that accompanies increased albumin synthesis may increase the risk of cardiovascular disease.

TABLE 3–4.
Common Causes of the Nephrotic Syndrome

Primary glomerular disease
Membranous nephropathy
Focal segmental glomerular sclerosis
Minimal change nephropathy
Membranoproliferative GN
Secondary glomerular disease
Diabetic nephropathy
Amyloidosis
Lupus nephritis

Hematuria and Proteinuria

Hematuria and proteinuria together usually imply the presence of glomerular inflammation; however, mild to moderate amounts of each can be seen in interstitial nephritis, or a chronic proteinuric state may have a superimposed cause of nonglomerular hematuria (see the separate proteinuria and hematuria sections). Clues that are very suggestive of glomerular disease are urinary protein greater than 3 gm/day and RBC casts.

The syndrome of acute GN includes the findings of edema, hematuria, and hypertension with proteinuria, urinary RBC casts, and diminished glomerular filtration rate. The prototype is post-streptococcal GN, which generally does not necessitate renal biopsy if the diagnosis is clear cut and the course unremarkable. Under most circumstances, however, such syndromes will require biopsy, because histology will influence therapeutic decision making.

A diagnostic workup would usually proceed as outlined in the proteinuria section; though, a fulminant course may necessitate immediate biopsy. A convenient method for limiting differential diagnosis is based on serum complement levels, with the cautions that those disorders usually presenting with low complements may not always have low complements and that hereditary complement deficiencies may be misleading (Table 3–5).

End-Stage Renal Disease, Dialysis, and Transplantation

Definitions

Dialysis.—movement of solutes down a concentration gradient across a semipermeable membrane

Ultrafiltration.—hydraulic or osmotic pressure-forced movement of liquid and solutes across a semipermeable membrane

End-Stage Renal Disease

End-stage renal failure, or disease (ESRD), can be defined as a persistent state of reduced renal function at less than 10% of normal, implying fewer than 10% of nephrons remain functional. Equivalently, the GFR, the measure of renal function, is less than 10 ml/minute.

The progression to ESRD is typically gradual and predictable; the reciprocal of the serum creatinine can be plotted against time

TABLE 3–5.
Causes of Hematuria and Proteinuria

	C3	C4
Low complement		
Lupus erythematosus	Low	Low
Poststreptococcal GN	Low	Normal
Membranoproliferative GN		
Type I	Normal or decreased	Normal or decreased
Type II	Normal or decreased	Normal or decreased
Cryoglobulinemia	Low	Low
Endocarditis	Low	Low
Normal complement		
Vasculitis		
IgA nephropathy		
Focal segmental glomerular sclerosis		
Goodpasture's syndrome		
Interstitial nephritis		
Hereditary nephritis		
Hemolytic uremic syndrome and thrombotic thrombocytopenic purpura		

and a linear extrapolation drawn to a predicted onset of renal failure. Over time, should the slope of the line change to become more negative, suggesting a more rapid deterioration of renal function, a reason should be sought and the problem alleviated.

Medical management considerations in each phase of the progression to ESRD are outlined in Table 3–6. The most common causes of ESRD are listed in Table 3–7. Specific treatment modalities, dialysis, and transplantation, are discussed below.

TABLE 3–6.
Clinically Relevant Considerations of the Metabolic Consequences of Renal Insufficiency

---

I. Glomerular filtration rate less than 100 ml/minute, and greater than 20 m/l minute
   A. Search for reversible causes.
   B. Control hypertension
   C. Treat hyperphosphatemia with oral phosphate binders.
   D. Adjust dosage of renally cleared drugs and avoid nephrotoxic drugs.
II. Glomerular filtration rate less than 20 ml/minute, and greater than 5 ml/minute
   A. Refer to I.
   B. Restrict potassium, sodium, and protein generally to 2, 2, and 60 gm/day, respectively.
   C. Consider fluid restriction if necessary.
   D. Document extent of renal osteodystrophy with hand and clavicle radiographs, parathyroid hormone level.
   E. Supplement calcium and vitamin D.
   F. Plan for maintenance dialysis and consider transplantation.
III. Glomerular filtration rate less than 5 ml/minute
   A. Refer to I and II.
   B. Initiate dialysis.

TABLE 3–7.
Common Causes of End-Stage Renal Disease

---

1. Glomerulonephritis
2. Hypertension
3. Polycystic kidney disease
4. Interstitial nephritis
5. Diabetes mellitus
6. Hereditary nephritis

Dialysis and Transplantation (Table 3–8)

TABLE 3–8.
Indications for Dialysis

1.	Acidosis
2.	Electrolyte abnormalities, particularly hyperkalemia
3.	Fluid overload
4.	Uremic symptoms (nausea, emesis, pruritis, lethargy, etc.)
5.	Drug toxicities and ingestions

Dialysis

Hemodialysis

Blood is pumped from a large vascular access at flow rates of 150 to 300 ml/minute through a semipermeable membrane. Dialysate fluid flows in an opposite direction and under lesser pressure, achieving a combination of dialysis and ultrafiltration.

High blood flow rates and the consequent efficiency of hemodialysis (HD) make it best suited for treating emergencies like hyperkalemia and drug toxicities (e.g., barbiturates, methanol, and lithium) and should be used in patients who can tolerate fluctuations in blood pressure (i.e., hypertensives without symptomatic coronary artery disease).

Problems related to rapid clearance rates include hypotension and rapid fluid and electrolyte shifts, which can result in the disequilibrium syndrome; a self-limited postdialysis syndrome manifested as headaches, vomiting, confusion, seizures, and coma.

Maintenance HD can usually be accomplished in three, 3- to 4-hour dialysis sessions per week. Long-term HD may result in dialysis dementia, characterized by myoclonus and progressive dementia believed to be due to excessive aluminum accumulation. Achieving vascular access and maintaining it free from infection and thrombosis can become limiting and even life-threatening factors.

Peritoneal Dialysis

A dialysate fluid made hypertonic with glucose is infused into the peritoneal cavity, where diffusion of solutes occurs across the semipermeable peritoneal surfaces. Ultrafiltration also occurs as

TABLE 3–9.
Peritoneal Dialysis Dialysate Composition

Solute		mEq/L	Milliosmoles/L
Sodium		132	132
Calcium		3.5	1.7
Magnesium		1.5	0.7
Chloride		102	102
Lactate		35	35
Glucose	1.5%		83
	4.25%		236
Totals	1.5%		355
	4.25%		508

the hypertonic solution draws fluid from the peritoneal micro-vasculature.

Peritoneal dialysis (PD) is a much slower process than HD and requires considerably longer dialysis times. A patient may be completely independent and ambulatory during dialysis with continuous ambulatory PD (CAPD), and would be less likely to suffer the effects of rapid fluid and electrolyte shifts.

Fluid removal with instillation of hypertonic fluid (from 1.5%-4.25% glucose) occurs rapidly initially, then decreases exponentially; most occurs in the first 30 minutes, and beyond 4 hours, fluid is slowly reabsorbed. Fluid removal and dialysis can be hastened with frequent short-duration dwells. Alternatively, fluid removal can be increased over a standard dwell time by increasing the glucose concentration of dialysate, though dialysis efficiency is not remarkably improved.

Hypokalemia may be prevented by adding 3.5 mEq/L to dialysate. Though these hypertonic glucose solutions may cause hyperglycemia, regular insulin can be added to PD fluid, which may even suffice for diabetic control. Maintenance CAPD can be achieved with three daily 5- to 6-hour dwells and one overnight dwell 7 days/week.

Peritoneal dialysis requires much patient compliance, meticulousness, and dexterity, but even under the best circumstances bouts of peritonitis may occur. Peritonitis is defined by a PD fluid leukocyte count of 100/cu mm or greater with 50% neutrophils. The most common causative organisms are skin flora, staphylococci, and streptococci; *Enterobacteriaceae* may be skin flora as well but suggest a break in bowel wall integrity. Minimally symptomatic patients without gram-negative infection may be managed as outpatients with intraperitoneal (IP) antibiotics. After full IV loading doses, maintenance IP antibiotic dosing can be accomplished by making the IP drug concentration the same as the desired blood level.

Continuous Arteriovenous Hemofiltration

A shunt is created by cannulating the femoral artery and vein and placing a semipermeable membrane (artificial kidney) between the two. Arterial pressure alone forces blood through the membrane and ultrafiltration occurs. A negative pressure on the ultrafiltrate side is created by maintaining a fluid-filled column from the kidney apparatus to a collecting bag suspended below. Ultrafiltrate is discarded and replaced with electrolyte balanced solutions. This technique is ideal for volume-overloaded patients in a critical care setting who may not tolerate hemodynamic instability; drawbacks are its invasive nature and exsanguination risk should a connection fail.

Transplantation

Clearly, many inherent problems with dialytic therapy can be overcome by implanting a viable kidney in a patient with renal failure. Immunosuppressive therapy, particularly cyclosporine, and human lymphocyte antigen typing have been responsible for improved patient and graft survival rates. Unfortunately, altered cell-mediated immunity makes these patients susceptible to cytomegalovirus, pneumocystis, *Listeria*, *Nocardia*, and *Aspergillus* infections.

Transplant rejection, typically manifested as progressive renal insufficiency and a tender renal graft, is difficult to distinguish from the reversible renal insufficiency of cyclosporine toxicity. This may require a therapeutic trial of immunosuppressive agents or graft biopsy to guide therapy.

FLUID AND ELECTROLYTES

Hyperkalemia

Definition

Hyperkalemia = a serum potassium concentration greater than 5.5 mEq/L

General Concepts

The various causes of hyperkalemia can be categorized into four main groups. Redistribution refers to a net migration of potassium ions from the intracellular fluid (ICF) to the ECF. The most common example of this phenomenon is seen in acidosis. The second category, decreased renal excretion, can occur through a number of mechanisms and represents the leading cause of hyperkalemia. Increased intake of potassium almost never causes hyperkalemia with normal renal function. It should be noted that cell lysis syndromes are most often responsible for the extreme cases of hyperkalemia that require emergency therapy. Pseudo-hyperkalemia occurs when the measured serum potassium concentration is greater than the patient's true serum potassium concentration. An ECG is often helpful in distinguishing pseudohyperkalemia from true hyperkalemia.

Causes of Hyperkalemia

  I. Redistribution (ICF → ECF)
     A. Cell lysis: rhabdomyolysis, tumor lysis, hemolysis, burns
     B. Acidosis (inorganic)
     C. Insulin deficiency
     D. Hyperosmolar state
     E. Drugs: succinylcholine, β-adrenergic antagonists, and nonsteroidal anti-inflammatory drugs
     F. Familial periodic paralysis

 II. Decreased renal excretion
     A. Renal insufficiency: acute renal failure, oliguric chronic renal failure, and chronic interstitial nephritis

    B. Mineralocorticoid deficiency: Addison's disease, hyporeninemic hypoaldosteronism, heparin

    C. Tubulointerstitial disorders: type IV renal tubular acidosis (RTA), system lupus erythematosus, sickle cell disease, amyloidosis, obstructive nephropathy, and renal transplants

    D. Potassium sparing diuretics: spironolactone, triamterene, and amiloride

    E. Angiotensin-converting enzyme inhibitors

    F. Nonsteroidal antiinflammatory agents

III. Increased intake
    A. Potassium replacement therapy
    B. Salt substitutes
    C. Hemolyzed blood transfusions
    D. Potassium salts of antibiotics

IV. Pseudohyperkalemia
    A. Thrombocytosis (platelet count $> 10^6$)
    B. Leukocytosis (WBC $> 70K$)
    C. In vitro hemolysis
    D. Venous sampling with tourniquet

Manifestations of Hyperkalemia (Table 3–10)

TABLE 3–10.
Hyperkalemia Manifestations

Neuromuscular Effects	Cardiac Effects	Hormonal Effects
Weakness	ECG abnormalities (see ECG changes)	Adrenal ↑ Aldosterone ↑ Epinephrine
Areflexia	Ventricular arrhythmia	Renal ↑ Renin
Paralysis	Cardiac arrest	Pancreas ↓ Glucagon ↑ Insulin

Electrocardiogram Changes in Hyperkalemia

1. Tall, narrow, peaked T-waves (esp. precordial leads)
2. ST segment elevation
3. Decreased amplitude of R-wave
4. Widened QRS complex
5. Prolonged P-R interval
6. Decreased amplitude or disappearance of P-wave
7. QRS complex merges with T-wave to form sine wave pattern

Therapy for Hyperkalemia

Before specific therapy is determined, it is helpful to classify hyperkalemia according to severity. Mild hyperkalemia refers to a serum potassium concentration less than 6.5 mEq/L and ECG changes limited to peaking of the T-waves. Moderate hyperkalemia is a serum potassium concentration of 6.5 to 8.0 mEq/L and ECG changes limited to peaking of the T-waves. Severe hyperkalemia is defined as a serum potassium concentration greater than 8.0 mEq/L or more advanced ECG changes.

When one is faced with hyperkalemia of any degree, several initial measures should be taken. Continuous ECG monitoring is always advisable, especially if the resting 12-lead ECG shows changes consistent with hyperkalemia. All potassium supplements, salt substitutes, and antibiotics containing potassium should be discontinued. Also, drugs that inhibit potassium excretion or promote redistribution (ICF → ECF) should be stopped. Finally, pseudohyperkalemia should be ruled out. This is relatively simple since most clinical chemistry laboratories will report significant in vitro hemolysis, and review of the patient's hematologic parameters will reveal thrombocytosis or leukocytosis. It may be necessary to obtain a repeat venous sample paying careful attention to correct venipuncture technique. Femoral vein sampling may be advisable because it does not involve a tourniquet.

Mild hyperkalemia may respond to these initial measures, but moderate to severe hyperkalemia should always be treated aggressively. There are essentially three ways to treat hyperkalemia. The first is to antagonize the neuromuscular and cardiac effects of hyperkalemia. In severe, life-threatening hyperkalemia, IV calcium should be given immediately. The beneficial effect takes place within minutes but lasts less than 1 hour, so other modalities will be necessary. The second is to shift the extracellular potassium to the intracellular compartment, and the third is to increase the excretion of potassium.*

Initial Measures for All Cases of Hyperkalemia

1. Obtain a 12-lead ECG.
2. Cardiac monitor.
3. Discontinue potassium supplements, salt substitutes, and potassium salt antibiotics.
4. Discontinue potassium-sparing diuretics and drugs that cause ICF → ECF shift.
5. Rule out pseudohyperkalemia.

Specific Therapy for Moderate to Severe Hyperkalemia

I. Antagonize effects of potassium: Administer 10 ml (1 amp) of 10% calcium gluconate intravenously over 2 to 4 minutes with ECG monitor. Repeat once in 5 minutes if the ECG changes persist.

II. Shift potassium (K^+) from ECF to ICF.
  A. Administer 500 ml of 10% glucose (10% aqueous dextrose solution, or $D_{10}W$) intravenously over 30 to 60 minutes, plus give 10 units of regular insulin subcutaneously. Or, administer 50 ml (1 amp) of 50% glucose ($D_{50}W$) intravenously over 5 minutes plus 10 units of regular insulin intravenously.
  B. Administer 50 ml (1 amp) of 7.5% sodium bicarbonate ($NaHCO_3$) intravenously over 5 minutes. Repeat in 15 minutes if ECG changes persist. Or, add 100 ml of 7.5% $NaHCO_3$ (2 amps) to 1,000 ml of $D_{10}W$ or $D_5\cdot9$ NaCl. Administer intravenously over 3 to 4 hours, plus give 25 units of regular insulin subcutaneously concurrently.

III. Excrete K^+
  A. Administer 20 to 40 gm of sodium polystyrene sulfonate (Kayexelate) in 50 to 100 ml of 20% sorbitol

---

*These measures have their onset of action within 1 hour, and the effects last for several hours.

orally or administer 30 to 50 gm of sodium polystyrene sulfonate in 100 to 200 ml of 20% sorbitol by
retention enema.
B. Perform hemodialysis or peritoneal dialysis.
C. Administer furosemide (Lasix) to the volume-overloaded patient.

HYPOKALEMIA

Definition

Hypokalemia = a serum potassium level less than 3.5 mEq/L.

General Concepts

The principal causes of hypokalemia can be categorized into three
groups. Redistribution refers to a net migration of potassium ions
from the ECF to the ICF. The most common example of this
phenomenon is seen in respiratory or metabolic alkalosis. Decreased intake of potassium is another means by which hypokalemia can occur. It may take several days to weeks before
inadequate potassium intake becomes clinically apparent. Increased excretion of potassium most commonly arises from two
sites, the GI tract and the kidney. Because urinary potassium is
usually a result of tubular secretion, most of the clinically important disorders associated with increased renal excretion of potassium are related to increased delivery of fluid to the distal
nephron, as seen with loop diuretics, increased mineralocorticoid
activity, or both.

Causes of Hypokalemia

  I. Redistribution (ECF → ICF)
     A. Alkalosis
     B. Treatment of hyperglycemia
     C. Hypokalemic periodic paralysis
 II. Decreased intake
     A. Alcoholism
     B. Anorexia nervosa
     C. Dietary indiscretions
III. Increased excretion

A. Gastrointestinal losses
  1. Diarrhea
     a. Laxative abuse
     b. Villous adenoma
  2. Ureterosigmoidostomy
B. Urinary losses
  1. Increased mineralocorticoid effect: primary hyperaldosteronism (Conn's syndrome), secondary hyperaldosteronism, Bartter's syndrome, increased glucocorticoid (Cushing's syndrome), licorice abuse (glycyrrhizic acid), and increased ACTH level
  2. Renal tubular acidosis (proximal and distal)
  3. Osmotic diuresis
  4. Alkalosis
  5. Increased excretion of poorly reabsorbed anion (lactic acidosis, ketoacidosis, and penicillins)
  6. Magnesium deficiency
  7. Amphotericin therapy
  8. Leukemias (lysozymuria)
  9. Diuretics
  10. Nasogastric suction/emesis

Manifestations of Hypokalemia

I. Neuromuscular: weakness, hyporeflexia, parethesias, paralysis, ileus, autonomic insufficiency, rhabdomyolysis, and worsening of hepatic encephalopathy

II. Cardiac: myocardial cell necrosis, atrial and ventricular arrhythmias, increased digitalis sensitivity, and ECG changes (see later discussion)

III. Renal: polyuria/polydipsia, decreased GFR, increased renal ammonia production, and hypokalemic nephropathy

IV. Hormonal: decreased aldosterone secretion and decreased insulin secretion

Electrocardiogram Changes of Hypokalemia
  1. ST segment depression
  2. Decreased T-wave amplitude

3. Prominent U-waves
4. Widened QRS complex
5. Increased amplitude and duration of P-wave
6. Arrhythmias (paroxysmal atrial tachycardia with block; 1st-, 2nd-, and 3rd-degree atrioventricular block, ventricular premature contractions, ventricular tachycardia, and ventricular fibrillation)

Therapy for Hypokalemia

Because of the potentially serious cardiac and neuromuscular sequelae, hypokalemia should be corrected immediately. An ECG is usually appropriate and should always be obtained when the serum potassium concentration is less than 2.5 mEq/L. Immediate IV replacement is required if cardiac arrhythmias, extreme muscle weakness, or respiratory distress occur. In life-threatening situations, up to 40 mEq/hour can be infused with continuous ECG monitoring. It should be recognized that rapid infusions of large amounts of potassium can be quite dangerous, and serum potassium determinations should be obtained frequently. In less critical situations, up to 10 mEq/hour can be safely administered intravenously without ECG monitoring.

The preferred means of potassium replacement is oral. Several different preparations, including liquids, effervescent tablets, and slow release tablets, are available. Infrequently, ulceration of the GI tract has been reported with the slow-release tablets, so liquid formulations are preferred. Several potassium salts, including potassium chloride, bicarbonate, citrate, and gluconate, are available. Potassium chloride is the salt of choice, except in the treatment of hypokalemia associated with metabolic acidosis (i.e., RTA). In these situations, potassium bicarbonate or bicarbonate equivalent (citrate or gluconate) is indicated. If there is concurrent hypophosphatemia, potassium phosphate should be used.

The amount of potassium to be replaced is difficult to estimate, and frequent serum potassium levels should generally be obtained during the period of replacement. However, rough guidelines for estimating the potassium deficit do exist. For example, in a 70-kg man, a decrease in serum potassium concentration from 4.0 to 3.0 mEq/L reflects a total body potassium deficit of 100 to 200 mEq. Below a serum potassium level of 3.0 mEq/L, each 1.0 mEq/L decrease represents an additional potassium deficit of

TABLE 3–11.
Hypernatremia Causes

Total body Na$^+$ Deficit (H$_2$O deficit > Na$^+$ deficit)	Normal Total Body Sodium Level (H$_2$O Deficit Only)	Total Body Sodium Excess (Na$^+$ > Excess H$_2$O)
Profuse sweating	Nephrogenic or central diabetes insipidus	Most commonly inappropriate administration of saline, sodium bicarbonate, etc.
Diarrhea		
Osmotic diuresis (i.e., urea, glucose, mannitol)		

200 to 400 mEq. Potassium replacement should be markedly reduced in patients with renal failure.

HYPERNATREMIA

Definition

Hypernatremia—a serum sodium determination greater than 145 mEq/L.

General Concepts

Hypernatremia reflects a deficit of free water relative to total body sodium:

Classify hypernatremia according to the total body sodium status, either low, normal, or increased. Deficits of sodium and water with relatively greater losses of water are classified as hypernatremia with low total body sodium. Loss of free water without loss of sodium results in hypernatremia with normal total body sodium. An absolute excess of sodium can cause hypernatremia with increased total body water, but this is uncommon.

Manifestations of Hypernatremia

Symptoms include thirst, restlessness, irritability, muscle twitching, and tremulousness. Signs include lethargy, obtundation, seizures, coma, hyperreflexia, and ataxia.

Therapy for Hypernatremia

The goal of treatment is restoration of a normal serum sodium level. The specific therapy depends primarily on the ECF volume status (sodium status). With low total body Na^+ levels, volume depletion may be clinically important (i.e., tachycardia, hypotension), and initial treatment should consist of IV infusion of isotonic 0.9% NaCl. When the patient is hemodynamically stable, treatment with D5.45% NaCl or D_5W may be instituted. With normal total body sodium the treatment is to replace the free water deficit. The volume of water required for adequate replacement can be estimated by calculating the free water deficit. In the setting of hypernatremia with increased total body sodium, treatment should be aimed at elimination of the excess sodium. This can be accomplished through the use of diuretics and replacement with water.

Free Water Deficit

Total body water (TBW) level $= 0.6 \times$ current body weight (kg)

$$\text{Desired TBW} = \frac{\text{Measured serum } Na^+ \times \text{current TBW}}{140}$$

Free water deficit $=$ desired TBW $-$ current TBW

Example: 70-kg man with serum $Na^+ = 155$.

Current TBW $= 0.6 \times 70$ kg $= 42$ L

$$\text{Desired TBW} = \frac{(155 \text{ mEq/L})(42 \text{ L})}{140 \text{ mEq/L}} = 46.5 \text{ L}$$

Free water deficit $= 46.5$ L $- 42$ L $= 4.5$ L.

NOTE: It is extremely important not to replace the entire deficit too quickly since this may result in cerebral edema and serious neurologic sequelae. It is advisable to replace no more than one half of the deficit in the first 12 to 24 hours. Frequent assessments of serum sodium levels and ECF volume are essential.

HYPONATREMIA

Definition

Hyponatremia $=$ a serum sodium concentration less than 135 mEq/L.

TABLE 3–12.
Causes of Hyponatremia

↓ Total Body Na+ (Euvolemic)	Normal (or Mildly ↓) Total Body Na+ (Normal or Slightly ↑ ECF Volume)	↑ Total Body Na+ Level (↑↑ ECF Volume)	Pseudohyponatremia
Diuretics	Hypothyroidism Drugs SIADH*	Nephrotic syndrome Cirrhosis Congestive heart failure Renal failure	Hyperlipidemia Hyperglycemia Hyperproteinemia

*Syndrome of inappropriate antidiuretic hormone secretion.

General Concepts

Hyponatremia reflects an excess of water relative to total body sodium. This is usually accompanied by decreased plasma osmolality. Hyponatremia may be associated with decreased, normal, or increased amounts of total body sodium (Table 3–12). Because sodium content is the principal determinant of ECF volume, these three categories are associated with decreased, normal or only mildly elevated, and elevated ECF volumes, respectively. The elevated ECF volume associated with the third category is manifest as edema.

Causes of Hyponatremia

An additional issue is that of hyponatremia with normal plasma osmolality, or *pseudohyponatremia*. This is seen with *hyperlipidemia* and *hyperproteinemia*. Hyponatremia with increased plasma osmolality reflects the presence of a large amount of another osmotically active solute in the ECF, such as glucose, ethanol, methanol, ethylene glycol, and mannitol.

Manifestations of Hyponatremia

Signs include abnormal sensorium, hyporeflexia, Cheynes-Stokes respirations, hypothermia, pseudobulbar palsy, and seizures. Symptoms include apathy, lethargy, disorientation, muscle cramps, anorexia, nausea, and agitation.

The severity of signs and symptoms depends not only on the serum sodium concentration but also on the rate of decrease. The more rapid the decline, the more severe the manifestations. Signs and symptoms are rare above serum sodium concentrations of 125 mEq/L.

Syndrome of Inappropriate Antidiuretic Hormone Secretion

Diagnostic Criteria
1. Hyponatremia with decreased plasma osmolality
2. Less than maximally dilute urine (usually >200 mOsm/dl)
3. No evidence of hypovolemia or edema
4. Normal renal, adrenal, and thyroid function
5. Absence of drugs that may impair water excretion
6. Absence of diuretics
7. Exclusion of other causes of hyponatremia

Antidiuretic Drugs
1. Nicotine
2. Morphine
3. Barbiturates
4. Clofibrate
5. Chlorpropamide
6. Tolbutamide
7. Cyclophosphamide
8. Vincristine
9. Acetaminophen
10. Indomethacin
11. Carbamazepine
12. Haloperiodol
13. Amitriptyline
14. Isoproterenol

Disorders Associated With the Syndrome of Inappropriate Antidiuretic Hormone Secretion

I. Carcinomas: lung (especially small cell), duodenum, and pancreas

II. Pulmonary disease: pneumonias, lung abscess, and tuberculosis

III. Central nervous system disease: encephalitis, meningitis, acute psychosis, stroke, intracranial bleed, brain tumor, brain abscess, head trauma, acute intermittent porphyria, and Guillain-Barrè syndrome

Therapy for Hyponatremia

Treatment of hyponatremia is guided by the clinical status of the patient as well as by the etiology of the disorder. Hyponatremia with a decreased total body sodium level is most appropriately treated by replacement of the ECF volume with normal saline and treatment of the underlying disorder. Hyponatremia with an increased total body sodium is best treated by initiation of water restriction, often in conjunction with diuretics. Again, proper management of the underlying disorder is essential. The therapy for hyponatremia with normal (or mildly increased) total body sodium level consists of correcting endocrine disorders such as hypothyroidism and glucocorticord deficiency and treatment of SIADH if present. Strict water restriction is the initial step in the management of SIADH. This often requires a relatively severe restriction of 500 to 1,000 ml of water/day. If this is not successful, 300 to 600 mg of demeclocycline should be administerd by mouth twice daily. Demeclocycline is contraindicated in liver disease.

Severe hyponatremia (Na^+ < 110 mEq/L) of any etiology is potentially life threatening and should be treated aggressively. Initial management should consist of water restriction, diuresis with a loop diuretic (furosemide, ethacrynic acid) and fluid replacement with normal saline.

Symptomatic hyponatremia (lethargy, disorientation, seizure, or coma) is a medical emergency and requires immediate treatment. In addition to water restriction and diuresis as previously mentioned, cautious use of hypertonic saline (3% NaCl) is indicated. The serum sodium concentration should be checked every 2 to 4 hours and should not be increased more rapidly than 1 mEq/hour. Hypertonic saline should no longer be used when the serum sodium concentration is more than 125 mEq/L. There have been reports of central pontine myelinolysis (CPM) following rapid correction of symptomatic hyponatremia with hypertonic saline, but the risks are believed to be less than those of persistent symptomatic hyponatremia. The use of hypertonic saline is particularly dangerous in patients with preexisting volume overload (renal failure, congestive heart failure, etc.) and should be used with extreme caution.

ACID-BASE DISORDERS

All acid-base disorders can be defined in terms of changes in pH, serum bicarbonate (HCO_3), and alveolar partial pressure of carbon dioxide ($PaCO_2$). Normal pH is 7.40 (± 0.04), HCO_3 is 24 (± 4) mEq/L, $PaCO_2$ is 40 (± 4) mm Hg.

There are four basic acid-base disorders: (1) metabolic acidosis, (2) metabolic alkalosis, (3) respiratory acidosis, and (4) respiratory alkalosis. Simple metabolic acidosis and alkalosis are characterized by $\downarrow$ pH, $\downarrow$ HCO_3 and $\uparrow$ pH, $\uparrow$ HCO_3, respectively. Compensatory changes of alveolar ventilation, and thus $PaCO_2$, occur to minimize changes in pH. Simple respiratory acidosis and alkalosis are characterized by $\downarrow$ pH, $\uparrow$ $PaCO_2$ and $\uparrow$ pH, and $\downarrow$ $PaCO_2$, respectively. Compensatory changes of renally controlled HCO_3^- excretion or regeneration occur to minimize changes in pH. It is important to note that over compensation does not occur.

The acid-base disorders are important for several reasons, including their direct effects on cardiovascular and central nervous systems, as well as reflecting underlying disease processes.

Arterial blood gas (ABG) measurements are essential to diagnose and interpret acid-base imbalances. An ABG measurement will provide values for pH, $PaCO_2$, and HCO_3^-. Samples should be obtained from an artery into a syringe coated with heparin. Air bubbles should be expelled and the sample placed in ice.

Interpretation of an ABG measurement involves knowledge of the clinical presentation of the patient and the chronicity of the patient's disorder, both of which can be readily obtained from the history and physical examination. Multiple clinical and experimental data in humans have been collected and can be summarized in the following nomogram (Fig 3–1).

One should note that the shaded areas represent "95% confidence" bands for the predicted acid-base disorders. If one obtains a sample falling outside the shaded areas, a mixed acid-base disorder must be suspected.

In acute respiratory acidosis or alkalosis, the degree of change expected is determined by the following expression:

$$10 \text{ mm Hg PaCO}_2 = \text{pH } .08.$$

For example, if the $PaCO_2$ equals 60 mm Hg, the change from the normal $PaCO_2$ is (60 mm Hg − 40 mm Hg), which is 20 mm Hg. The expected pH would be decreased by 0.16, or (7.40 − 0.16), which equals 7.24. If the actual measured pH varies from the expected pH by more than 0.02, one must suspect a metabolic component to the acid-base disorder, namely, a mixed acid-base disorder.

Metabolic Acidosis

Definition

Metabolic acidosis = a clinical condition causing a pH less than 7.35, HCO_3 less than 20 mEq/L, and a compensatory decrease in $PaCO_2$.

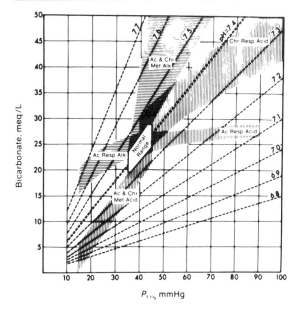

FIG 3–1

In vivo nomogram showing bands for uncomplicated respiratory or metabolic acid-base disturbances. Each confidence band represents the mean $\pm$ 2 SD for the compensatory response of normal subjects or patients to a given primary disorder. (From Braunwald E, Isselbacher KJ, Petersdorf RG, et al (eds): *Harrison's Principles of Internal Medicine*, ed 11. New York, McGraw-Hill Book Co, 1987. Used by permission.)

General Concepts

The formula

$$PaCO_2 = (1.0 - 1.5)\,(\Delta HCO_3)$$

reflects the degree of respiratory compensation expected. Clinically, metabolic acidosis is broken down into normal and increased anion gap (AG):

$$AG = [Na^+] - [(Cl^-) + (HCO_3^-)].$$

A normal AG is 8 to 12 mEq/L. A high AG is more than 12 mEq/L and usually indicates that a metabolic acidosis is present. Metabolic acidosis can be present with either high or normal AGs. In the high AG group, the increment in the AG should equal the decrement in HCO_3 from normal. In fact, when the decrement in HCO_3 is greater than the increment in AG, a mixed high AG and hyperchloremic acidosis exists. The opposite situation ($\Delta AG > \Delta HCO_3$) indicates a mixed metabolic alkalosis and metabolic acidosis.[2] Low AGs of less than 8 mEq/L may reflect disorders such as IgG multiple myeloma, hyperkalemia, hypercalcemia, hypermagnesemia, hypoalbuminemia, lithium intoxication, or laboratory errors secondary to methodology, such as low sodium levels with highly viscous serum and high chloride levels with bromide intoxication.

Causes of High Anion Gap Metabolic Acidosis
1. Renal failure
2. Diabetic ketoacidosis
3. Lactic acidosis
4. Alcoholic ketoacidosis
5. Starvation ketoacidosis
6. Salicylate intoxication
7. Ethylene glycol ingestion
8. Paraldehyde ingestion
9. Methanol ingestion

Causes of Normal Anion Gap Metabolic Acidosis
Hyperchloremic Acidosis

I. Bicarbonate loss
   A. Gastrointestinal: diarrhea, small bowel, biliary or pancreatic drainage, ureteral diversions, and anion exchange resins
   B. Renal: proximal (type II) RTA and dilutional acidosis

II. Failure of bicarbonate regeneration
   A. Renal: distal (type I) RTA, ingestion of acidifying salts and hyperalimentation

Manifestations of Metabolic Acidosis

I. Cardiovascular
   A. Depressed myocardial contractility
   B. Decreased peripheral vascular resistance
   C. Hypotension
   D. Ventricular fibrillation

II. Central nervous system
   A. Confusion
   B. Lethargy
   C. Coma

III. Pulmonary
   A. Hyperventilation with Kussmaul's respirations
   B. Pulmonary vasoconstriction
   C. Enhanced tissue oxygen delivery

IV. Electrolytes
   A. Increased extracellular potassium level (especially with mineral acidosis)
   B. Increased ionized calcium level

V. Gastrointestinal
   A. Emesis

Therapy for Metabolic Acidosis

In general, correction of the underlying cause is essential. Bicarbonate therapy is indicated when the pH is less than 7.15 or HCO_3 level is less than 10 mEq/L, although this is controversial in lactic acidosis and diabetic ketoacidosis. One's goal with bicarbonate therapy is to raise the pH to more than 7.20. The amount of bicarbonate needed is readily calculated by the following formula:

HCO_3 deficit = 0.5 × kg of body weight × (desired HCO_3 − measured HCO_3).

Each ampule of sodium bicarbonate contains 50 mEq. If the

blood pH is less than 7.10, one should substitute 0.8 for 0.5 in the formula given. The complications of therapy include volume overload, hypokalemia, hypocalcemia, overshoot alkalemia, and hyperosmolarity. Therefore, bicarbonate replacement should be cautiously administered. With chronic metabolic acidosis, as occurs in RTA and renal failure, oral repletion of bicarbonate is useful. Shohl's solution with sodium and/or potassium citrate contains 1 mEq/ml of solution. Metabolism of citrate generates bicarbonate.[3]

Metabolic Alkalosis

Definition

Metabolic alkalosis = a clinical condition causing a pH of more than 7.45, HCO_3 more than 28 mEq/L, and a compensatory increase in $PaCO_2$.

General Concepts

The formula, compensated $PaCO_2$ = baseline $PaCO_2$ + $(0.25 - 1.0)(\Delta HCO_3^-)$ reflects the degree of respiratory compensation expected. Clinically, metabolic alkalosis is broken down into two main categories: (1) Associated with NaCl and ECF depletion (urinary chloride [UCl] < 10 mEq/L), and (2) not associated with NaCl and ECF depletion (UCl > 20 mEq/L). The most important measurement to narrow the differential involves assessment of the urinary chloride at least 12 hours after diuretic use.

Causes of Saline- and Volume-Responsive Metabolic Alkalosis (UCl < 10 mEq/L)

I. Gastrointestinal
   A. Vomiting
   B. Nasogastric suction
   C. Villous adenoma
   D. Chloride diarrhea

II. Renal
   A. Diuretics
   B. Impermeant anion administration

III. Exogenous alkalosis
   A. Alkali administration
   B. Milk-alkali syndrome
   C. Blood transfusions

Causes of Saline- and Volume-Resistant Metabolic Alkalosis (UCl > 20 mEq/L)

 I. Mineralicorticoid excess
   A. Hyperaldosteronism
   B. Cushing's syndrome
   C. Bartter's syndrome
   D. Excess licorice intake
   E. Excess chewing tobacco
   F. Carbenoxolone ingestion
   G. Liddle's syndrome

 II. Profound potassium depletion

 III. Nonparathyroid hypercalcemia

 IV. Refeeding

 V. Hypoparathyroidism

Manifestations of Metabolic Alkalosis

 I. Cardiovascular
   A. Positive inotropy
   B. Arrhythmias especially if pH is more than 7.6

 II. Neuromuscular
   A. Paresthesias
   B. Twitching
   C. Cramping
   D. Laryngeal spasm
   E. Seizures
   F. Coma
   G. Positive Chvostek's and Trousseau's signs

 III. Electrolytes
   A. Hypokalemia
   B. Decreased ionized calcium
   C. Mild hypophosphatemia

Therapy for Metabolic Alkalosis

In general, correction of the underlying disorder is essential. Therapy diverges dramatically depending on the differential of saline-responsive and saline-resistant metabolic alkalosis.

   Saline-responsive metabolic alkalosis responds to volume repletion with IV normal saline. Potassium should also be repleted.

Removal of causative agents is essential.

Saline-resistant metabolic alkalosis requires removal of excess mineralocorticoid effect. This can be accomplished via removal or ablation of secretory tumors or via inhibition with spironolactone. Potassium repletion is necessary.

Respiratory Acidosis

Definition

Respiratory acidosis = a clinical condition causing a pH less than 7.35, $PaCO_2$ more than 45 mm Hg, and an elevated serum bicarbonate level that varies depending on the chronicity of the disorder.

General Concepts

Compensation is more complete with time, so that by 3 to 5 days full compensation is to be expected. The following formulas quantify the degree of renal-mediated bicarbonate compensation:

1. Acute ($<$ 24 hours), compensated HCO_3 = Baseline HCO_3 increases 1 mEq for every 10 mm Hg $PaCO_2$ increase
2. Chronic ($>$ 3–5 days), compensated HCO_3 = Baseline HCO_3 increases 4 mEq for every 10 mm Hg $PaCO_2$ increase

The underlying disorder here is alveolar hypoventilation. Alveolar hypoventilation is secondary to either decreased minute ventilation or ventilation-perfusion mismatches.

Causes of Respiratory Acidosis

I. Neuromuscular and central nervous system disorders
   A. Guillain-Barrè syndrome
   B. Myasthenia gravis
   C. Botulism
   D. Narcotic, sedative, or tranquilizer overdose
   E. Poliomyelitis
   F. Muscular dystrophy
   G. Brain stem injury
   H. Cerebrovascular accident
   I. General anesthesia

    J. Hypokalemia

    K. Myxedema

II. Airway obstruction

    A. Aspiration

    B. Bronchospasm or laryngospasm

    C. Laryngeal edema

    D. Chronic obstructive pulmonary disease

III. Decreased ventilation

    A. Pneumonia

    B. Pulmonary edema

    C. Adult respiratory distress syndrome

    D. Flail chest or kyphoscoliosis

IV. Miscellaneous

    A. Pulmonary embolism

    B. Cardiopulmonary arrest

    C. Ventilator malfunction

Manifestations of Respiratory Acidosis

I. Central nervous system

    A. Depression

    B. Anxiety

    C. Confusion

    D. Lethargy

    E. Delirium

    F. Headache

II. Neuromuscular

    A. Tremors

    B. Muscle jerks

    C. Clonic movements

    D. Weakness

III. Cardiovascular

    A. Decreased myocardial contractility

    B. Peripheral vasodilation

    C. Cor pulmonale

    D. Cardiac dysrhythmias

Therapy for Respiratory Acidosis

Correction of underlying disorders is essential. The key to therapy
is to *increase alveolar ventilation*. Alveolar ventilation can be

increased by reversing bronchoconstriction with bronchodilators such as β-adrenergic agonists, theophylline, or atrophine-like agents. Improved airway management via chest physical therapy, suctioning or endotracheal intubation with mechanical ventilation may be needed. Oxygen therapy may be required to maintain the PaO_2 more than 50 mm Hg. Sodium bicarbonate therapy is needed rarely.

Respiratory Alkalosis

Definition

Respiratory alkalosis = a clinical condition causing a pH more than 7.45, pCO_2 less than 35 mm Hg, and a decreased serum bicarbonate level that varies depending on the chronicity of the disorder.

General Concepts

As with respiratory acidosis, renal compensation can be expected to be complete by 3 to 5 days. The following formulas quantify the degree of change in bicarbonate compensation:

1. Acute (< 24 hours), compensated HCO_3 = Baseline HCO_3 decreases 1–3 mEq for every 10 mm Hg decrement in $PaCO_2$.
2. Chronic (> 3–5 days), compensated HCO_3 = Baseline HCO_3 decreases 2–5 mEq for every 10 mm Hg decrement in $PaCO_2$.

The underlying disorder here is alveolar hyperventilation. Alveolar hyperventilation may be stimulated by three different broad mechanisms: (1) central nervous system, (2) peripheral, and (3) miscellaneous.

Causes of Respiratory Alkalosis

I. Central nervous system
  A. Anxiety
  B. Cerebrovascular accident
  C. Head trauma
  D. Salicylates
  E. Fever
  F. Pain

      G. Pregnancy or progesterone

      H. Brain tumor

  II. Peripheral stimulation

      A. Pneumonia

      B. Congestive heart failure

      C. Pulmonary emboli

      D. Hypoxia

      E. Interstitial lung disease

      F. High altitude

  III. Miscellaneous

      A. Gram-negative sepsis

      B. Ventilator malfunction

      C. Hepatic insufficiency

      D. Hyperthyroidism

Manifestations of Respiratory Alkalosis

  I. Pulmonary

      A. Increased tidal volume

      B. Increased respiratory rate

  II. Neurologic

      A. Lightheadedness

      B. Muscle cramps

      C. Distal extremity paresthesias

      D. Tremor

      E. Circumoral paresthesias

      F. Tetany with positive Chvostek's sign

      G. Trousseau's sign

      H. Convulsions

  III. Cardiovascular

      A. Palpitations

      B. Atrial and ventricular arrhythmias

Therapy for Respiratory Alkalosis

Again, correction of the underlying disorder is essential. The key to therapy is to decrease alveolar ventilation.

BIBLIOGRAPHY

Hematuria and Proteinuria

Fairley KF, Birch DF: Hematuria: A simple method for identifying glomerular bleeding. *Kidney Int* 1982; 21:105–108.
Glassock RJ, Adler SG, Ward HJ, et al: Primary glomerular diseases and secondary glomerular diseases, Chapters 22 and 23, in Brenner BM, Rector FC (eds): *The Kidney*, ed 3. Philadelphia, WB Saunders Co, 1986, vol 1.

Acute Renal Failure

Miller TR, et al: Urinary indices in acute renal failure. *Ann Intern Med* 1978; 89:47–50.

Hematuria

Bullock N: Asymptomatic microscopical haematuria. *Br Med J* 1986; 292:645.
Copley JB: Review: Isolated asymptomatic hematuria in the adult. *Am J Med Sci* 1986; 291:101–111.

Proteinuria

Abuelo JG: Proteinuria: Diagnostic principles and procedures. *Ann Intern Med* 1983; 98:186–191.
Lewis EJ: Proteinuria, in Stein JH (ed): *Internal Medicine*. Boston, Little, Brown & Co, 1983, pp 674–676.

Hematuria and Proteinuria

Fairley KF, Birch DF: Hematuria: A simple method for identifying glomerular bleeding. *Kidney Int* 1982; 21:105–108.
Glassock RJ, Adler SG, Ward HJ, et al: Primary glomerular diseases and secondary glomerular diseases, Chapters 22 and 23, in Brenner BM, Rector FC (eds): *The Kidney*, ed 3. Philadelphia, WB Saunders Co, 1986, vol 1.

Chronic Renal Failure, Dialysis and Transplantation

Alfrey AC: Chronic renal failure: Manifestations and pathogenesis, in Schrier RW (ed): *Renal and Electrolyte Disorders*. Boston, Little, Brown & Co, 1986, pp 461–494.
Klahr S: Chronic renal failure, in Stein JH (ed): *Internal Medicine*. Boston, Little, Brown & Co, 1983, pp 690–700.

Levey AS, Harrington JT: Continuous peritoneal dialysis for chronic renal failure. *Medicine* (Baltimore) 1982; 61:330–339.

Manis T, Friedman EA: Dialytic therapy for reversible uremia. *N Engl J Med* 1979; 301:1260–1265, 1321–1328.

Nolph KD, Whittier FC: Treatment of chronic renal failure, in Stein JH (ed): *Internal Medicine*. Boston, Little, Brown & Co, 1983, pp 806–815.

Peterson PK, Andersen RC: Infection in renal transplant recipients. *Am J Med* 1986; 81(suppl 1A):2–10.

Popovich RP, et al: Continuous ambulatory peritoneal dialysis. *Ann Intern Med* 1978; 88:449–456.

Fluid and Electrolytes

Berl T, Anderson RJ, McDonald KM, et al: Clinical disorders of water metabolism. *Kidney Int* 1976; 10:117.

Gennari JF: Serum osmolality. *N Engl J Med* 1984; 310:102.

Narins RG, Jones ER, Stone MC, et al: Diagnostic strategies in disorders of fluid, electrolyte and acid-base homeostasis. *Am J Med* 1982; 72:496.

Bidani A: Electrolyte and acid-base disorders. *Med Clin North Am* 1986; 70:1013.

Goldberg M: Hyponatremia. *Med Clin North Am* 1981; 65:251.

Schrier RW: *Renal and Electrolyte Disorders*. Boston, Little, Brown & Co, 1980.

Chou TC: *Electrocardiography in Clinical Practice*. New York, Grune & Stratton, 1979.

Emmett M, Narins RG: Clinical use of the anion gap. *Medicine* (Baltimore) 1977; 56:38–54.

Goodkin DA, Krishna GG, Narins RG: The role of the anion gap in detecting and managing mixed metabolic acid-base disorders. *Clin Endocrinol Metab* 1984; 13(2):339-349.

Schrier RW: *Renal and Electrolyte Disorders*, ed 3. Boston, Little, Brown & Co, 1986, pp 141–206.

Seldin DW, Rector FC Jr: The generation and maintenance of metabolic alkalosis. *Kidney Int* 1972; 1:306–321.

Stein JH: American College of Physicians, Medical Knowledge Self-assessment. Program VII, 1986, pp 494–498.

Wyngaarden JB, Smith LH Jr: *Cecil Textbook of Medicine*, ed 17. Philadelphia, WB Saunders Co, 1985.

Cardiology

R. Jeffrey Snell, M.D.
Scott Adelman, M.D.

A 12-lead electrocardiogram (ECG) is an imperative diagnostic tool when evaluating any patient with a cardiac disturbance. It is of utmost importance to properly examine and interpret a 12-lead ECG.

ECGs AND DYSRHYTHMIAS*

I. Complexes and intervals
  A. p waves: p waves normally are upright in leads 1, 2, AVF, and V4–6; inverted in AVR, and variable in lead 3, AVL, and other chest leads.
  Abnormalities:
    1. Inversion of p waves can be seen when the impulse travels through the atria via an abnormal pathway (e.g., ectopic atrial or atrioventricular nodal rhythms).
    2. Increased amplitude usually indicates atrial hypertrophy or dilation.
    3. Increased width usually indicates atrial enlargement or diseased atrial muscle. Normal p waves do not exceed 0.11 seconds in duration. With a diphasic, wide p wave in lead V1, a broad inverted terminal component suggests left atrial enlargement.
    4. Notching may be present when the left atrium is enlarged (e.g., mitral disease). The p wave becomes widened and notched and is taller in lead 1 than lead 3; this is called p-mitrale.
    5. Peaking indicates overload of the right atrium (e.g., chronic obstructive pulmonary disease)

*Adapted from Marriott HJ: *Practical Electrocardiography,* ed 8. Baltimore, Williams & Wilkins, 1988.

and produces pointed p waves that are taller in lead 3 than lead 1; this is called p-pulmonale.

B. P-R interval (normal = 0.12 to 0.20 seconds).

1. Shortened (<0.12 seconds).

   a. Atrioventricular (AV) and junctional and low atrial rhythms.

   b. Bypass tracts: Wolff-Parkinson-White syndrome, Lown-Ganong-Levine syndrome.

   c. Glycogen storage disease.

   d. Normal variant.

2. Prolonged (>0.20 seconds).

   a. Coronary artery disease, rheumatic heart disease, hyperthyroidismrare.

   b. Drugs, digoxin, β-blockers, verapamil.

   c. Normal variant.

C. Q-T interval.

Corrected Q-T (Q-T$_c$) (normal ≤0.44) =
$$\frac{\text{Q-T interval (seconds)}}{\sqrt{\text{R-R interval (seconds)}}}$$

1. A shortened Q-T interval can be seen with digitalis, hyperkalemia, hypercalcemia, acidosis, and hyperthyroidism.

2. A prolonged Q-T interval can be seen with congenital abnormalities, ischemic heart disease, hypothermia, cardiomyopathy, mitral valve prolapse, heart block, and cerebral lesions (especially subarachnoid hemorrhage), electrolyte disorders (hypokalemia, hypocalcemia), and drug effects (especially quinidine, procainamide, phenothiazines).

II. Axis (Fig 4–1).

A. Causes of axis deviation:

1. Right axis deviation. Normal variant. Mechanical shifts: inspiration, emphysema. Right ventricular hypertrophy. Right bundle branch block. Dextrocardia. Wolff-Parkinson-White syndrome.

2. Left axis deviation. Normal variant. Mechanical shifts: expiration, high diaphram from pregnancy, ascites, etc. Left bundle branch block.

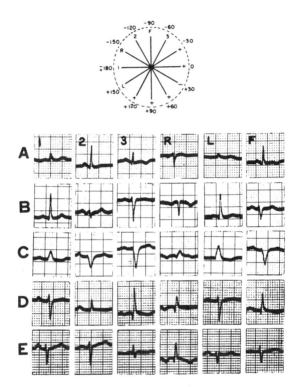

FIG 4–1

ECG leads illustrating axes in the frontal plane. The QRS axis in each tracing is as follows: $A = +60°$; $B = -30°$; $C = -70°$; $D = +135°$; $E = -135°$. (From Marriott HJL (ed): *Practical Electrocardiography,* ed 8. Baltimore, Williams & Wilkins Co, 1987. Used by permission.)

Congenital heart disease. Wolff-Parkinson-White syndrome.

III. Chamber enlargement.
 A. Left ventricular hypertrophy (LVH). Voltage criteria: add depth of S-wave in V1 to height of R wave in V5 or V6 (whichever is taller). LVH is present if the sum is greater than 35 mm. Supporting criteria include: LAD and QRS prolongation.

The most common cause is hypertension. It is also seen in aortic valve disease, coarctation of the aorta, and hypertrophic cardiomyopathy.

 B. Right ventricular hypertrophy (RVH).
  1. R:S ratio in V1 > 1.0 (reversal of precordial pattern).
  2. QRS width is within normal limits.
  3. Right axis deviation.
  4. ST depression with upward convexity and inverted T wave in V1–2.

Common causes include congenital heart disease (e.g., tetralogy of Fallot, pulmonic stenosis, transposition of the great vessels), valvular lesions such as mitral stenosis and tricuspid insufficiency, and chronic lung disease.

IV. Bundle branch block (BBB).
 A. Complete BBB, QRS ≥0.12 (Table 4–1).
 B. Fascicular blocks:
  1. Criteria for left anterior fascicular block (LAFB):
   a. Left axis deviation (usually > −30°).
   b. Small Q in I and AVL; small R in 2, 3, AVF.

TABLE 4–1.
Bundle Branch Block

Lead	LBBB	RBBB
V1	QS or RS	RSR¹ (biphasic variant), sometimes wide R or qR (monophasic variant)
V6	No Q waves, monophasic R	Wide S wave
1	Monophasic R, no Q	Wide S wave

    2. Criteria for left posterior fascicular block
      (LPFB):
      a. Right axis deviation (usually $> +\ 120°$).
      b. Small S in lead I and AVL; small Q in 2,
        3, AVF.
      c. No evidence of RVH.

V. Specific dysrhythmias.
  A. Sinus tachycardia.
    Definition: Increased rate of discharge of the sinus
    node (> 100 beats per minute), which may be sec-
    ondary to multiple factors (e.g., exercise, fever,
    anxiety, pain, hypovolemia) and which represents a
    physiologic response to a demand for increased car-
    diac output.
    Treatment: Treat underlying process.
  B. Sinus bradycardia.
    Definition: Slowing of the sinus node discharge rate
    to less than 60 beats per minute, which may be due
    to intrinsic sinus node disease, increased parasym-
    pathetic tone, or drug effects.
    Treatment: Unnecessary unless hypotension or ven-
    tricular ectopic beats are present at which time atro-
    pine is the drug of choice. A transvenous pacemaker
    may be necessary.
  C. Premature atrial complexes (PACs).
    Definition: An electrical impulse which originates in
    the atria outside the sinus node. It is premature and
    characterized by a non-compensating pause (the in-
    terval between the sinus P wave preceding and fol-
    lowing the PAC is less than twice the normal P-P
    interval).
    Clinical: It can be a normal variant or it can be
    caused by factors such as stimulants (e.g., caffeine,
    tobacco), sympathomimetic drugs (e.g., inhaled
    bronchodilators), hypoxia, or congestive heart fail-
    ure.
    Treatment: Usually unnecessary or directed at the
    underlying cause. Occasionally quinidine, procain-
    amide, a β-blocker, or digitalis can be used.

D. Atrial tachycardias.

Definition: A rhythm with a rate greater than 100 beats per minute that originates in the atria outside the sinus node usually due to re-entry or increased automaticity. P waves when present have a different appearance from sinus P waves, and the QRS complexes are usually narrow.

1. Paroxysmal atrial tachycardia (PAT) or PAT with block has features described above but also frequently has associated AV block and an abrupt onset and termination. It may be a manifestation of digitalis toxicity.

2. Multifocal atrial tachycardia (MAT) is also as above but is characterized by at least three different P wave appearances, each with a specific P-R interval.

   Clinical: These rhythms are usually seen with structural heart disease and atrial enlargement. Other causes include alcohol intoxication, chronic obstructive pulmonary disease, and acute myocardial infarction. MAT is usually associated with underlying pulmonary disease.

   Treatment: The underlying cause should be treated. Digitalis, verapamil, or β-blockers can be used to control the ventricular response. Quinidine or procainamide can be used to try to convert the dysrhythmia back to sinus rhythm. In PAT, digitalis should be withheld from the patient and hypokalemia corrected. MAT is notoriously refractory to therapy.

E. Atrioventricular reentrant tachycardia.

Definition: A regular tachycardia at 110 to 250 beats per minute usually initiated by a PAC and usually with a narrow QRS. Most commonly reentry is via the AV node. Patients may present with syncope, palpitations, or chest pain.

Treatment: Depends on the stability of the hemodynamics. If the patient is hypotensive, cardioversion with DC countershock should be attempted. Vagal maneuvers frequently terminate the tachycardia in the hemodynamically stable patient. The drug of choice is intravenous verapamil. Intravenous digitalis or β-blockers may also be effective.

F. Atrial fibrillation and flutter.

Definition: Lack of organized atrial electrical activity leading to ineffective atrial contractions. Discrete P-waves are absent and small F waves are substituted. Usual AV conduction is at about 100 to 180 beats per minute in patients with normal AV node function. Classically, the ventricular response is irregularly irregular. Atrial flutter is characterized by flutter waves, which give the pathognomonic saw tooth appearance to the ECG. In untreated patients, AV nodal conduction is usually 2:1 in atrial flutter giving a ventricular response that is regular, usually at a rate of 150 beats per minute.

Clinical: either rhythm can be chronic or episodic. Chronic atrial fibrillation is usually related to organic heart disease or valvular heart disease with atrial dilatation. Other causes of either chronic or paroxysmal atrial fibrillation include: hypertensive heart disease, diminished left ventricular function, thyrotoxicosis, pericarditis, pulmonary embolism, or after cardiac surgery.

Atrial flutter is usually unstable either reverting to normal sinus rhythm or progressing to atrial fibrillation. Treatment: Due to a loss of atrial ventricular synchrony, there is a decrease in cardiac output. In some patients this is well tolerated while in others this may lead to hemodynamic collapse. Treatment will depend on the clinical circumstance. If the patient is hypotensive, DC countershock is the treatment of choice (25 to 50 joules for flutter; 50 to 100 joules for fibrillation). Medical treatment is directed at controlling the ventricular rate. Intravenous digoxin, verapamil, or β-blockers are effective. Once the ventricular response is controlled, oral quinidine or procainamide can be used in an attempt to convert the arrhythmia back to normal sinus rhythm.

G. Junctional tachycardia.

Definition: Due to an increased rate of a junctional pacemaker. ECG shows a regular rhythm with a QRS of a similar appearance as supraventricular beats. There may or may not be retrograde conduction to the atria. The P wave may occur before, during, or after the QRS complex.

Clinical: Usually seen in either acute myocardial infarction or digitalis toxicity.

Treatment: Usually no acute treatment is necessary.

H. Premature ventricular complex (PVC).

Definition: An ectopic impulse arising prematurely in the ventricle either due to re-entry or enhanced automaticity. The altered sequence of ventricular activation results in a wide bizarre QRS and abnormal ST-T changes. Since the rhythmicity of the sinus node is not usually disturbed, a full compensatory pause results.

Clinical: May be a normal variant with frequency increasing with age. In ischemic heart disease, the frequency of PVCs and incidence of sudden death increase with a decrease in ventricular function.

Treatment: When PVCs occur infrequently in a patient without other suspicion of heart disease, therapy is generally unnecessary. For acute suppression, lidocaine is the drug of choice with procainamide and bretylium being secondary agents. Many drugs can be used for chronic oral therapy including procainamide, quinidine, disopyramide, mexilitine, etc.

I. Ventricular tachycardia (VT).

Definition: Three or more ventricular complexes in succession with a rate greater than 100 beats per minute. Sustained VT lasts longer than 30 seconds and causes hemodynamic instability. Differentiating VT from SVT with aberrancy can be difficult. Factors suggestive of VT include: AV dissociation, the presence of fusion beats, a QRS duration greater than 0.14 seconds, a monophasic or biphasic RBBB complex in V1 (rather than the usually triphasic

RSR′ complex), and left axis deviation in the frontal plane.

Clinical: Can be seen in ischemic heart disease, CHF, secondary to drug effects, hypokalemia, and hypomagnesemia. A greater incidence and mortality is seen in ischemic heart disease and after a myocardial infarction.

Treatment: Acute therapy includes DC countershock if the patient is hemodynamically compromised and lidocaine or procainamide if stable. Many drugs exist for chronic oral therapy as listed under PVCs. All have a potential proarrhythmic effect. For patients with potentially lethal VT, electrophysiologic studies (EPS) are suggested. A noninducible VT during EPS supports effective anti-arrhythmic therapy. Those in whom drug therapy fails after multiple attempts may be candidates for an automatic implantable defibrillator (AID).

J. Ventricular fibrillation.

Definition: A chaotic ventricular rhythm without organized ventricular depolarization or contraction associated with hemodynamic instability.

Treatment: DC countershock should be attempted as soon as possible. As long as no effective thythm is present, cardiopulmonary resuscitation (CPR) should be performed. Epinephrine, lidocaine, and bretylium should be given in sequence to facilitate defibrillation.

K. Asystole.

Definition: Absence of electrical activity.

Treatment: CPR must be initiated. Intravenous epinephrine and atropine should be used. Sodium bicarbonate, isoproterenol, and calcium chloride may occasionally be useful. A ventricular pacemaker may be beneficial.

L. Atrioventricular block (AV block).

1. First-degree AV block.

Definition: Delay in passage of the impulse from atria to ventricles characterized by a P-R

interval greater than 0.20 seconds.
Treatment: None indicated.

2. Second-degree AV block, type I (Wenckebach).
   Definition: A progressive decrement in conduction almost always at the AV node level characterized by three features: group beating, progressive P-R prolongation, and progressive decrement in the R-R interval. This abnormality can be caused by increased parasympathetic tone or drug effect (e.g., digitalis, β-blockers). Therapy: This rhythm is often transient and carries a favorable prognosis. If the ventricular rate becomes excessively slow, atropine is usually effective. A pacemaker is seldom necessary.

3. Second-degree AV block, type II.
   Definition: This block usually occurs below the AV node and is characterized by dropped beats without a preceding P-R prolongation. It is unusual for more than one non-conducted beat to occur in succession.
   This rhythm is due to an organic lesion in the conduction pathway and is not the result of increased parasympathetic tone or drug effect; hence, it carries a worse prognosis.
   Treatment: A temporary pacemaker is necessary until a permanent pacemaker can be inserted.

4. Third-degree AV block.
   Definition: The complete absence of conduction between the atria and ventricles that may occur with the block at or below the AV node. The escape rhythm may either be junctional or ventricular.
   Treatment: When the block occurs at the level of the AV node, atropine may be effective, otherwise a pacemaker is required.

HEART FAILURE

I. Acute congestive heart failure begins precipitously and is

not well tolerated. Chronic congestive heart failure elic-
its several physiologic compensations including increased
sympathetic tone, redistribution of blood flow, and an
increased renin-angiotensin-aldosterone axis.

II. Left and right heart failure. Left ventricular (LV) failure
   is the most common cause of right ventricular (RV) failure, but disorders that cause RV failure such as pulmonary hypertension, pulmonary/tricuspid valve disease,
   and right ventricular infarction should always be kept in
   mind.

III. Low vs. high output failure. While low cardiac output
    characterizes most forms of heart failure, several high-
    output states including thyrotoxicosis, beri-beri, Paget's
    disease of bone, anemia, and pregnancy should be con-
    sidered.

IV. Etiology: Longstanding hypertension, CAD, valvular disease, pericardial disease, toxins (adriamycin, alcohol),
   inflammatory disorders (infectious, collagen/vascular diseases), and infiltrative disorders (amyloid, sarcoid, hemochromatosis) should be considered in the differential
   diagnosis.

V. Precipitating factors:
   A. Noncompliance with diet and medications.
   B. Pulmonary emboli, acute myocardial infarction, and
      dysrhythmias.
   C. Drugs: cardiac depressants (B-blockers, calcium
      channel blockers, anti-arrhythmics), sodium-retain-
      ing drugs (steroids, nonsteroidal anti-inflammatory
      drugs).
   E. Increased metabolic demands (fever, activity, ane-
      mia, pregnancy, weight gain).

VI. Symptoms.
   A. LV failure: exertional dyspnea, orthopnea, paroxys-
      mal nocturnal dyspnea, dyspnea at rest, nocturia,
      acute pulmonary edema, angina, and hypoxia.
   B. RV failure: Dyspnea due to decreased cardiac output
      and underlying pulmonary parenchymal disease, diz-
      ziness, syncope secondary to decreased cardiac out-
      put, peripheral edema, anasarca.

C. New York Heart Association (NYHA) functional classification: class I: no limitations; class II: slight limitation, comfortable at rest but ordinary activity results in fatigue; class III: marked limitation, still comfortable at rest but less than ordinary activity causes symptoms; class IV: inability to carry on any activity without discomfort, symptoms even present at rest.

VII. Physical findings.

A. General: variable from normal to differing degrees of dyspnea due to cardiac cachexia and Cheyne-Stokes respirations.

B. Pulmonary: rales, wheezing, and pleural effusions.

C. Cardiovascular: jugular venous distension, pulsus alternans (advanced failure), maximal cardiac impulse displaced laterally, presence of an S3 and pronounced P2, and systolic murmurs secondary to mitral regurgitation or tricuspid regurgitation.

D. Abdomen: congestive hepatomegaly and ascites.

E. Extremities: edema and cyanosis are common.

VIII. Treatment.

A. General approach: two factors should be addressed in the management of congestive heart failure:

1. Removal of the underlying cause, which may require surgical correction of structural abnormalities such as congenital malformations and acquired valvular lesions. Medical treatment of conditions such as infective endocarditis or hypertension.

2. Control of the congestive heart failure state, which may be divided into three categories:

a. Improvement of cardiac performance with digitalis glycoside, sympathomimetic agents, other positive inotropes, or a pacemaker.

b. Reduction of workload with vasodilator therapy.

c. Control of excessive salt and water retention with a low sodium diet and fluid restriction, diuretics and mechanical removal of fluid (e.g., thoracentesis, paracentesis, dialysis, phlebotomy).

d. Dietary and lifestyle changes can be integrated with available pharmacologic agents into a treatment plan related to the patient's functional classification.

IX. Acute pulmonary edema (Cardiogenic).

A. Stages.

1. Stage I: Increased lymph flow without net gain of interstitial fluid, and decreased PO_2 with an increased A-a gradient.

2. Stage II: Interstitial edema: worsening tachypnea with deterioration in gas exchange, and inspiratory crackles on physical examination.

3. Stage III: Alveolar edema: tachypnea, sometimes frothy pink sputum, and severe hypoxemia. Chest x-ray shows greater density towards proximal hilar regions.

B. Therapy.

As with chronic forms of congestive heart failure, look for precipitating causes. Management is aided by Swan-Ganz catheterization.

1. Intravenous morphine, 2–5 mg repeated as necessary. This reduces anxiety and adrenergic vasoconstrictive stimuli.

2. Supplemental oxygen.

3. Intravenous loop diuretics, usually lasix, which also exerts a venodilator action initially.

4. Nitroglycerin to reduce preload.

5. Afterload reduction with intravenous nitroprusside, especially if arterial blood pressure is elevated.

6. Occasionally theophylline will be of value as a bronchodilator.

7. Rotating tourniquets or phlebotomy if the above therapy is unsuccessful.

CORONARY ARTERY DISEASE

I. Ischemic heart disease. Ischemia refers to a lack of oxygen due to inadequate perfusion. Ischemic heart disease has a diverse etiology having in common an imbalance between oxygen supply and demand.

  A. Etiology and pathophysiology.

     1. Causes of ischemia include: atherosclerosis of epicardial coronary arteries (most common); a decrease in coronary blood flow or secondary to arterial thrombi, spasm, arteritis; a marked increase in oxygen demand (e.g., left ventricular hypertrophy from hypertension or stenosis); a decrease in oxygen carrying capacity (e.g., severe anemia, carbon monoxide exposure).

     2. Atherosclerosis. The normal myocardium extracts a very high and relatively fixed percentage of oxygen. Atherosclerotic plaques, located in the large epicardial coronary arteries can severely limit the myocardial mechanism for increasing oxygen supply. A significant lesion is an obstruction of greater than 70% in one of the three main coronary arteries.

     3. Risk factors. Major: hypertension, smoking, diabetes mellitus, hypercholesterolemia, and a positive family history. Minor: age, sex, obesity, physical inactivity.

  B. Clinical manifestations.

     1. Asymptomatic disease: Atherosclerosis is a progressive disease, which often starts prior to the age of 20 years and remains asymptomatic for long periods with or without characteristic ECG changes.

     2. Sudden death: May be the initial manifestation in 33% of patients.

     3. Angina pectoris:

       a. Caused by transient myocardial ischemia.

       b. About 80% of patients with typical angina are men.

     c. Typical patients are 50- to 60-year-old men with troublesome or frightening chest discomfort, usually described as heaviness, pressure, squeezing, or smothering. The pain is usually substernal in location, occasionally radiating to the left shoulder, back, neck, or jaw. It is crescendo-decrescendo in quality and 1 to 5 minutes in duration.

     d. Frequently related to exercise, cold, or emotion but may occur at rest. Sharp fleeting chest pains or prolonged dull aches localized to the left inframammary region are rarely due to myocardial ischemia.

C. Diagnostic evaluation.

  1. History and risk factor assessment remain an integral starting point.

  2. While a normal resting ECG does not exclude ischemic heart disease, findings such as old myocardial infarction (MI) or repolarization abnormalities (ST-T changes) add suspicion. Typical ST and T wave changes that accompany episodes of angina and disappear thereafter are more specific. The ST segment is usually depressed during angina but may be elevated as in early MI or Prinzmetal's angina.

  3. Stress testing: standard protocols utilize incremental increases in external workload while vital signs and the ECG are continuously monitored. A positive test is greater than 1.0 mm ST depression 0.08 seconds beyond the J point (S-T junction). Other ECG changes, symptoms, blood pressure changes, and dysrhythmias are noted as well. A normal test is one in which the patient achieves the 85% predicted maximum heart rate for age and sex without ECG changes or symptoms. False-positive or false-negative results are about 10% and 30%, respectively. False-positive results are more common in women, patients on cardiac

drugs such as digitalis or quinidine, and in those with an abnormal resting ECG, especially with LVH or LBBB. Predictive accuracy can be improved in these patients by the addition of thallium to demonstrate reversible perfusion defects or an echocardiogram to demonstrate reversible wall motion abnormalities.

4. Coronary arteriography currently remains the gold standard for defining coronary anatomy. Indications include: patients with chronic stable or unstable angina in whom medical therapy is refractory or who are being considered for percutaneous transluminal coronary angioplasty or coronary artery bypass surgery (CABG); patients with atypical symptoms that present diagnostic difficulties to establish or rule out the diagnosis of coronary artery disease; patients suspected of having left main or severe three-vessel disease, regardless of symptoms; patients with aortic stenosis or hypertropic cardiomyopathy and angina; and most MI patients at high risk (e.g., recurrent angina, congestive heart failure or dysrhythmias).

D. Management.

1. Reduction of risk factors.
2. Elimination of coexistent illness.
3. Adaptation of activity.
4. Drug therapy (as delineated in formulary): nitrates, β-blockers, calcium channel blockers.
5. Mechanical revascularization.

   a. Percutaneous transluminal coronary angioplasty (PTCA) may be considered in patients with 1-, 2-, or occasionally 3-vessel disease and angina accompanied by evidence of ischemia on ECG. Patients with suitable proximal lesions in major coronary arteries, even if asymptomatic, are considered candidates by some centers. The overall mortality rate is less than 1%; the need for emergency CABG is 3% to 5%; and the risk of an MI is about 3%. Stenosis of an artery that perfuses a large area with poor collateral vessels and calcified plaques increases the risks. Adequate dilatation with relief of angina is achieved in 85% to 90% of patients. There is a 15% to 40% rate of restenosis within 6 months. If restenosis occurs, the success rate of repeat PTCA is slightly better than the first procedure.

b. Coronary artery bypass graft surgery: Clinical trials have defined the following points: mortality rates can be less than 1% in experienced hands, reocclusion occurs in 10% to 20% of vein grafts during the first year and 2% per year thereafter, angina is abolished or significantly decreased in 85% of patients. Mortality is reduced for patients with left main lesions, some reduction also occurs with three-vessel disease and reduced LV ejection fraction. There is no evidence that mortality is reduced in patients with one-vessel or two-vessel disease who have chronic stable angina and normal LV ejection fractions.

II. Unstable angina.
   A. Definition: Includes four groups of patients: those with angina of recent onset (less than 6 weeks) that is severe and frequent; those with angina of any duration that occurs at rest; those with chronic stable angina with a recent increase in intensity, frequency, or duration of pain; those with angina developing or becoming more severe within days or weeks of an acute MI.
   B. Management:
      1. Admit, preferably to a cardiac care unit and monitor.
      2. Recommend aggressive use of β-blockers, calcium-channel blockers, nitrates, aspirin, heparin, morphine, and oxygen.

      3. Intravenous nitroglycerin if persistent pain.

      4. Placement of an intra-aortic balloon pump if the above measures are unsuccessful.

      5. Cardiac catheterization is indicated for almost all patients with unstable angina. The incidence of significant left main lesions may be as high as 20%.

III. Myocardial infarction (MI). Approximately 1.5 million MIs occur per year. The mortality rate is about 35% with more than half of these deaths occurring within the first 2 hours after the onset of symptoms, usually due to malignant ventricular dysrhythmias. An additional 15% to 20% of patients die within 1 year.

  A. Diagnosis.

  Formally requires two of the following three criteria: characteristic history, evolutionary changes on ECG, and elevated cardiac enzymes (Fig 4–2).

  B. Management.

    1. *General measures*: bedrest, ECG monitoring, and oxygen therapy.

    2. *Pain control*: morphine sulfate, β-blockers, nitroglycerin (sublingual, paste, or continuous intravenous drip). If blood pressure becomes a limiting factor, an intra-aortic balloon pump may be indicated.

    3. *Reperfusion*: animal and human studies indicate that reperfusion improves hemodynamics, decreases infarct size, and promotes functional recovery if carried out within 4 hours and preferably within 2 hours of the onset of chest pain. Risk/benefit ratios appear best for anterior infarctions. Efficacy in clot lysis: intracoronary streptokinase = 70% to 80%; intravenous streptokinase = 50% to 70%; intravenous or intracoronary tissue plasminogen activator = 70% to 90%. Following successful thrombolysis, high-grade stenoses are frequent and may predispose to reocclusion and definitive procedures are usually required.

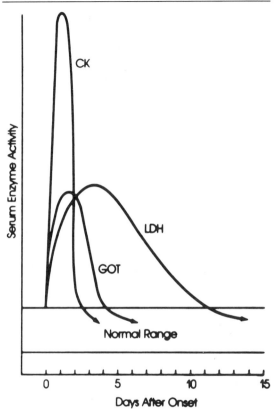

FIG 4–2

The time course of serum enzyme concentration changes following a typical myocardial infarction. *CK* = creatinine phosphokinase; *LDH* = lactic dehydrogenase; *GOT* = glutamic oxaloacetic transaminase. (From Braunwald E, Isselbacher KJ, Petersdorf RG, et al (eds): *Harrison's Principles of Medicine,* ed 11. New York, McGraw-Hill Book Co, 1987. Used by permission.)

4. *Anticoagulant therapy*: recent data suggest that patients with anterior wall myocardial infarctions are at a high risk (33%) for development of a mural thrombus, especially if apical hypokinesis occurs. Patients should undergo two-dimensional echocardiography and be treated with full-dose intravenous heparin if a thrombus is present.

5. *Rehabilitation*: patients with no complications should be progressively ambulated over 7 to 10 days of hospitalization. Low-level exercise testing prior to discharge permits identification of patients at increased risk for subsequent cardiac events.

C. Complications.

1. *Dysrhythmias*: See prior section for management.

2. *Congestive heart failure*: Management is facilitated with hemodynamic monitoring (Swan-Ganz, A-line). Four distinct subsets of patients can be identified and are categorized by the pulmonary capillary wedge pressure (PCWP) and cardiac index (CI) (Table 4–2).

3. Extension or recurrence occurs in 10% to 15% at 7 to 10 days.

4. Rupture of septum or papillary muscle may present as refractory congestive heart failure and a new loud holosystolic murmur. Medical therapy includes afterload reduction and IABP, but surgery is often required.

5. Right ventricular infarction is usually associated with a transmural inferior wall MI. Diagnosis is made with Swan-Ganz catheterization (increased RA pressure with normal PCWP; steep Y descent in the right atrial tracing, dip and plateau in the RV tracing). Treatment includes volume replacement with inotropic support. Diuretics are not indicated.

6. Pericarditis: Treat with nonsteroidal antiinflammatory drugs.

TABLE 4-2.
Classes of Congestive Heart Failure

Class	PCWP > 18 mmHg	CI <2.2 L/min/m²	Mortality Rate (%)	Therapy
I	−	−	3	As per uncomplicated MI (vide supra)
II	+	−	9	Diuretics; reduce afterload if blood pressure is elevated
III	−	+	23	Volume expansion
IV (cardiogenic shock)	+	+	51	Diuretics; afterload reduction as tolerated; inotropic support (dobutamine, dopamine); IABP

IV. Cardiomyopathies.
   A. Definition:
      This is a group of disorders characterized by dysfunction of the myocardium. They may be primary or secondary and do not include hypertensive cardiovascular disease, cor pulmonale, valvular heart disease, or congenital disorders. They may present with symptoms of congestive heart failure.
   B. Functional classification:
      1. Dilated congestive (D): LV dilated with decreased contractility.
      2. Restrictive (R): LV diastolic filling impairment.
      3. Hypertrophic (H): LV inappropriately hypertrophied often with asymptomatic septal hypertrophy, normally with preserved or hyperdynamic LV contractility, with or without obstruction to ventricular outflow.
   C. Etiologic classification:
      1. Primary: idiopathic (D,R,H), familial (D,H), eosinophilic endomyocardial disease (D,R), endomyocardial fibrosis (R).
      2. Secondary:
         a. Infective (D): viral, bacterial, fungal, protozoal.
         b. Metabolic (D).
         c. Familial storage disease (D,R): glycogen storage disease, mucopolysaccharidoses.
         d. Connective tissue diseases (D,R): systemic lupus erythematosus, polyarteritis nodosa, rheumatoid arthritis, scleroderma, dermatomyositis.
         e. Infiltrative/granulomatous (D,R): amyloid, sarcoid, malignancy, hemochromatosis.
         f. Neuromuscular (D): muscular dystrophy, myotonic dystrophy, Friedrich's ataxia, Refsum's disease.
         g. Toxic agents (D): alcohol, radiation, drugs.
         h. Peripartum heart disease (D).
   D. Treatment: Depends on the type of cardiomyopathy and a complete discussion is beyond the scope of this text.

ALGORITHMS

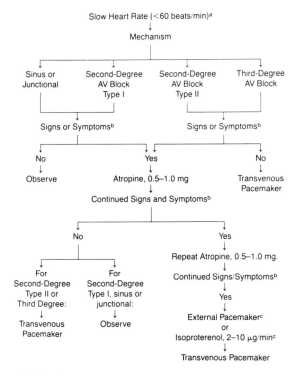

FIG 4–3
Algorithm for bradycardia. (From Jaffe AS, et al: *Textbook of Advanced Cardiac Life Support.* American Heart Association, 1987. Used by permission.)

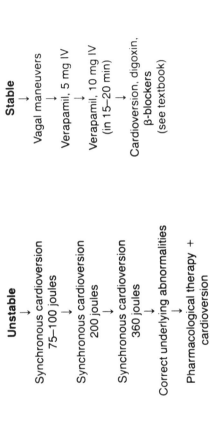

Unstable

Synchronous cardioversion
75–100 joules
→
Synchronous cardioversion
200 joules
→
Synchronous cardioversion
360 joules
→
Correct underlying abnormalities
→
Pharmacological therapy +
cardioversion

Stable

Vagal maneuvers
→
Verapamil, 5 mg IV
→
Verapamil, 10 mg IV
(in 15–20 min)
→
Cardioversion, digoxin,
β-blockers
(see textbook)

If conversion occurs but PSVT recurs, repeated electrical cardioversion is *not* indicated. Sedation should be used as time permits.

FIG 4–4
Algorithm for paroxysmal supraventricular tachycardia. (From Jaffe AS, et al: *Textbook of Advanced Cardiac Life Support.* American Heart Association, 1987. Used by permission.)

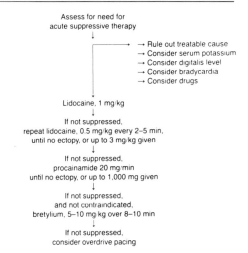

Once ectopy is resolved, maintain as follows:

After lidocaine, 1 mg/kg . . . . .Lidocaine drip, 2 mg/min
After lidocaine, 1–2 mg/kg . . . . .Lidocaine drip, 3 mg/min
After lidocaine, 2–3 mg/kg . . . . .Lidocaine drip, 4 mg/min
After procainamide . . . . .Procainamide drip, 1–4 mg/min
                                                              (Check blood level.)
After bretylium . . . . .Bretylium drip, 2 mg/min

FIG 4–5

Algorithm for ventricular ectopy. (From Jaffe AS, et al: *Textbook of Advanced Cardiac Life Support*. American Heart Association, 1987. Used by permission.)

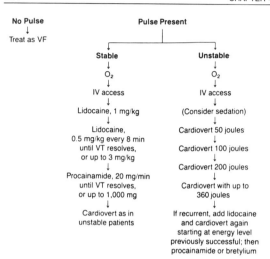

FIG 4–6

Algorithm for sustained ventricular tachycardia. (From Jaffe AS, et al: *Textbook of Advanced Cardiac Life Support.* American Heart Association, 1987. Used by permission.)

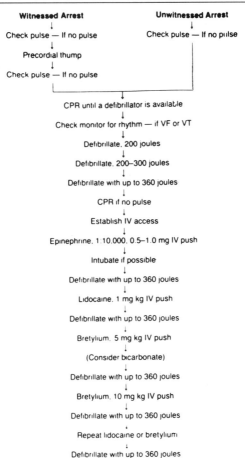

Witnessed Arrest
↓
Check pulse — If no pulse
↓
Precordial thump
↓
Check pulse — If no pulse

Unwitnessed Arrest
↓
Check pulse — If no pulse

CPR until a defibrillator is available
↓
Check monitor for rhythm — if VF or VT
↓
Defibrillate, 200 joules
↓
Defibrillate, 200–300 joules
↓
Defibrillate with up to 360 joules
↓
CPR if no pulse
↓
Establish IV access
↓
Epinephrine, 1:10,000, 0.5–1.0 mg IV push
↓
Intubate if possible
↓
Defibrillate with up to 360 joules
↓
Lidocaine, 1 mg/kg IV push
↓
Defibrillate with up to 360 joules
↓
Bretylium, 5 mg/kg IV push
↓
(Consider bicarbonate)
↓
Defibrillate with up to 360 joules
↓
Bretylium, 10 mg/kg IV push
↓
Defibrillate with up to 360 joules
↓
Repeat lidocaine or bretylium
↓
Defibrillate with up to 360 joules

FIG 4–7

Algorithm for cardiac arrhythmias in adults. (From Jaffe AS, et al: *Textbook of Advanced Cardiac Life Support.* American Heart Association, 1987. Used by permission.)

Asystole

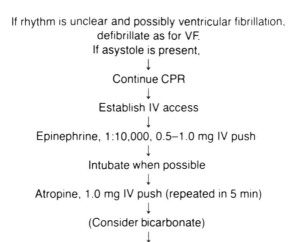

If rhythm is unclear and possibly ventricular fibrillation,
defibrillate as for VF.
If asystole is present,
↓
Continue CPR
↓
Establish IV access
↓
Epinephrine, 1:10,000, 0.5–1.0 mg IV push
↓
Intubate when possible
↓
Atropine, 1.0 mg IV push (repeated in 5 min)
↓
(Consider bicarbonate)
↓
Consider pacing

FIG 4–8
Algorithm for asystole.

BIBLIOGRAPHY

Braunwald E (ed): *Heart Disease—A Textbook of Cardiovascular Medicine*, ed 3. Philadelphia: Saunders Co, 1987.
Braunwald E, Isselbacher KJ, Petersdorf RG, et al (eds): *Harrison's: Principles of Internal Medicine*, ed 11. New York, McGraw-Hill Book Co, 1988.
Marriott, HJL (ed): *Practical Electrocardiography*, ed 8. Baltimore, Williams & Wilkins, 1987.

Gastroenterology and Hepatology

John Phelan, M.D.
Jeffrey Dugas, M.D.
William Hallmon, M.D.
Sheldon Sloan, M.D.
Peter Stein, M.D.

GASTROINTESTINAL BLEEDING

I. Pathophysiology of hypovolemia.
   A. Rapidity of blood loss may be a more important determinant than quantity in initial presentation.
   B. Mild blood loss is defined as a loss of 10% to 15% of intravascular volume.
      1. Volume is preserved by mobilizing extravascular reserves and contraction of venous vessels.
      2. Blood flow to the heart and brain are still preserved.
      3. With rapid bleeding, shock may develop even with only a 10% loss of blood volume.
   C. Moderate blood loss is defined as a loss of greater than 15% of volume.
      1. Heart rate and contractility increase and peripheral vasoconstriction occurs.
      2. Aldosterone and antidiuretic hormone (ADH) output increase.
      3. With decreased circulating volume and tissue hypoxia, lactic acidosis occurs.
      4. Respiratory rate is increased.

D. Severe blood loss is defined as a loss of greater than 30% of blood volume.

    1. Hypotension is always present.

    2. Diminished blood volume and cardiac output lead to poor oxygen delivery and end-organ damage. Acute renal failure, shock liver (massively elevated transaminase levels), and/or myocardial infarction may develop.

II. Assessment.

A. The characterization of bleeding.

    1. Melena is a black tar-like stool and suggests a minimum of 200 mL of blood lost above the ligament of Treitz.

    2. Hematemesis may be either bright red blood or coffee grounds material. Emesis without blood does not exclude an upper gastrointestinal (GI) source, since the bleeding may come from the duodenal bulb.

    3. Hemoccult testing of stool and vomitus is only useful if the material appears like it may be blood. Material not resembling blood should not be tested with hemoccult.

B. Vital signs.

    1. An orthostatic blood pressure drop of 10 mmHg implies a 10% to 20% loss of intravascular volume.

    2. Tachycardia and hypotension imply more than 30% loss of intravascular volume.

    3. An orthostatic pulse increase of greater than 10 beats per minute implies a greater than 10% loss of blood volume.

C. Nasogastric tube (NG).

    1. This is used primarily to determine upper GI bleeding. A return of grossly bloody material localizes the bleeding to the upper GI tract. A negative return does not exclude upper GI bleeding, since as many as 16% of such patients have been found to have bleeding lesions at endoscopy.

2. A 16 to 18 F tube is recommended.
3. Tap water is used to lavage the stomach of blood. Cold solutions are not any more efficacious over room temperature solutions and may interfere with coagulation.
4. There are almost *no* contraindications to NG tube passage, including esophageal varices.
5. Levarterenol 8 mg/100 mL passed via NG tube has not been proven beneficial.
6. Antacids via NG tube interfere with endoscopy and have not demonstrated efficacy in stopping bleeding. Histamine blockers will not stop bleeding, but may prevent future bleeding.

D. Physical examination.
1. Vital signs: see above.
2. Cutaneous manifestations of liver disease (spider angiomata, palmar erythema, gynecomastia, jaundice) may be associated with variceal bleeding.
3. Cardiac examination: aortic stenosis may be associated with angiodysplasia.
4. Neurologic examination: hepatic encephalopathy and asterixis may be seen in cirrhotic patients who have variceal or other sources of upper GI bleeding.
5. Abdominal examination: one should look for ascites and splenomegaly in cirrhotics. Peritoneal signs and a sudden loss of abdominal pain may suggest a perforated ulcer.
6. Rectal examination: one must look for bleeding hemorrhoids and check color (red or tar) and consistency of stool.

E. Laboratory tests.
1. SMA-6: elevated blood urea nitrogen (BUN) may be seen in upper GI bleeding. BUN and creatinine levels may be elevated in acute renal failure related to volume loss.
2. Hematocrit may be normal initially as it takes 6 to 8 hours to equilibrate after acute blood loss.

The hematocrit should be followed as frequently as every hour or less frequently depending on the rate of bleeding.

3. In active bleeding, platelets should be maintained >50,000/mm³.

4. Prothrombin time and partial thromboplastin time may be abnormal in cirrhosis and should be followed up and maintained with vitamin K or plasma to preserve hemostasis.

III. Intravascular replacement.
  A. The patient's blood should be typed and cross-matched for packed red blood cells or whole blood.
  B. Volume repletion should be guided by orthostatic vital signs, and normal saline as a bolus of 300–500 mL should be given if the patient has orthostasis.
  C. If the patient remains orthostatic after 1 L of saline, packed red blood cells should be transfused. This should be done sooner in patients for whom oxygen transport is critical (i.e., patients with coronary artery disease, chronic obstructive pulmonary disease, etc.).
  D. Other indicators of organ perfusion and oxygenation must also be monitored to guide therapy, including urine output, mental status, liver function tests, and cardiac monitoring. In patients in whom hemodynamic status is compromised by underlying congestive heart failure, central venous pressure monitoring via a Swan-Ganz catheter may be appropriate.
  E. Platelet transfusion should be used if more than 50% of volume is lost or if there is underlying thrombocytopenia.
  F. Fresh frozen plasma may be given in massive bleeding or in instances in which the patient presents with a prolonged prothrombin or partial thromboplastin time.

IV. Diagnostic intervention.
  A. Endoscopy.
    1. For life-threatening, continuous bleeding, en-

doscopy is indicated to plan definitive therapy (variceal sclerotherapy, surgery).

2. For patients who are easily stabilized without evidence of ongoing bleeding, endoscopy can be performed electively.

3. In patients in whom bleeding has ceased, a major benefit of endoscopy is to identify risk factors for re-bleeding (e.g., varices, visible vessels in an ulcer) and thus plan further intervention.

B. Angiography.

1. The procedure of choice in patients with massive lower GI bleeding.

2. Allows an opportunity for therapeutic intervention with embolization or vasopressin administration.

3. Able to detect bleeding rates of 0.5–1.0 mL/min.

C. ^{99m}Tc-labelled RBCs.
Useful for patients with chronic (subacute) bleeding in situations in which other diagnostic procedures have been unsuccessful.

D. Sigmoidoscopy/colonoscopy.

1. Useful in patients who have slower bleeding rates.

2. Allows for biopsy of polyp and/or polypectomy.

3. Cautery or laser therapy may be used to stop bleeding in certain situations (see below).

E. Barium studies.
No role in acute bleeding, particularly in the lower GI tract.

F. Anoscopy.
Used to detect hemorrhoidal bleeding.

G. Meckel's scan.
Technetium study that localizes ectopic parietal cells. Used in the diagnosis of bleeding of obscure origin in children and young adults.

V. Therapy.

A. Cautery/laser.

For nonvariceal bleeding, cautery and yttrium-aluminum-garnet lasers have been used. Cautery is effective in up to 90% of patients. Laser is expensive and has the potential to cause deep tissue burns or perforations.

B. Sclerotherapy for esophageal varices.

The American College of Physicians position paper advocates sclerotherapy for patients who are not surgical candidates or who are bleeding despite vasopression or balloon tamponade. Others use urgent sclerotherapy as the initial treatment in all patients.

C. Embolization with gelfoam or autologous clot.
1. Performed in patients who are poor surgical risks.
2. Useful for peptic ulcers, Mallory-Weiss tears, diverticular hemorrhage, and bleeding malignancies.
3. Complications include ischemic damage distal to the embolization site.

D. Vasopressin.
1. Used intravenously for variceal bleeding in conjunction with more definitive procedures (shunting, sclerotherapy). Given as a drip beginning at 0.3 U/min titrated up to a maximum of 1 U/min by 0.1 U/min increments at 30–60-min intervals.
2. Complications include coronary artery spasm and mesenteric ischemia for which nitroglycerin is often administered concomitantly.
3. Vasopressin will control bleeding in 40% to 70% of patients but does not favorably influence survival rates.

E. Shunt surgery (splenorenal, portacaval, mesocaval).
1. Allows decompression of varices.
2. Up to 90% effective in some series, particularly in nonalcoholics. Alcoholics have a much poorer outcome.
3. Operative mortality is 10% to 15%. Higher for patients in Child's class C.
4. Encephalopathy is a major cause of morbidity and mortality.

F. Pharmacotherapy.
   1. Histamine (H2) receptor blockade is routinely given but has no demonstrated efficacy in stopping acute episodes even when given in conjunction with antacids. Additionally, in critically ill patients, H2 receptor blockade has been shown to increase the rate of serious infections due to gram-negative bacteria and mortality when given prophylactically.
   2. Vasopressin (see above).
   3. Somatostatin decreases splanchnic blood flow and gastric acid secretion. Data on efficacy are still controversial.
   4. Prostaglandins are potent mesenteric vasoconstrictors. No data on efficacy are available at this time.

COLON CANCER AND POLYPS

I. Polyps.
   A. No malignant potential.
      1. Hyperplastic.
      2. Hamartomas found in Peutz-Jeghers and benign juvenile polyposis.
      3. Inflammatory pseudopolyps found in inflammatory bowel disease.
   B. Malignant potential: Adenomas.
      Premalignant nature is related to size.
      1. 1 cm: 1% to 2% malignant.
      2. 1–2 cm: 5% to 10% malignant.
      3. Greater than 2 cm: 10% to 40% malignant.
      4. Villous adenomas: highest malignant potential.

II. Surveillance for colon cancer.
   A. Average risk patient (age 40 to 50 years old).
      1. Yearly rectal examination with testing for occult blood.
      2. Two consecutive yearly flexible sigmoidoscopies beginning at age 50 years old. If normal, then every 3 to 5 years.
   B. Mildly increased risk.
      1. First degree relative with colon cancer.

      2. History of genitourinary or breast cancer.
         a. As in A., but beginning 5 to 10 years ear-
            lier than index case.
  C. Moderately increased risk.
     1. Prior colorectal cancer or adenoma.
     2. Family history of cancer family syndrome or
       breast cancer with colon cancer.
        a. Begin screening at age of diagnosis or age
          20 years.
        b. Yearly rectal examination with occult blood
          testing.
        c. Barium enema studies or colonoscopy every
          1 to 3 years after two normal yearly exami-
          nations.
  D. High-risk patients.
     1. Familial polyposis.
     2. Inflammatory bowel disease.
       a. Begin screening at age 10 to 20 years in po-
         lyposis syndromes or after 7 to 10 years of
         pancolitis.
       b. Yearly sigmoidoscopy with colonoscopy
         every 1 to 3 years.
       c. Biannual occult blood testing.

III. Colon cancer.
  A. Epidemiology.
     1. 57,000 deaths annually.
     2. Men and women equally affected.
     3. Location: 21% in cecum and ascending colon,
       22% in rectum, and 26% in descending colon
       and sigmoid.
  B. Presentation.
     1. Change in bowel habits and/or weight loss
       (signs of obstruction more frequent in lesions of
       left colon).
     2. Iron deficiency anemia.
     3. Tenesmus (rectal cancer).
     4. Occult blood in stool (more frequent in lesions
       in cecum and ascending colon).
  C. Diagnosis.
     1. Rectal examination detects 50%.

      2. Barium enema studies, colonoscopy (more sensitive).

      3. Carcinoembryonic antigen (CEA) levels are useful only for follow-up after resection, and are not to be used for screening or diagnostic purposes.

  D. Staging: Duke's classification.

Stage A: Invasion into the submucosa, no lymph nodes affected and no metastases.

Stage B: Invasion through the serosa, no lymph nodes affected and no metastases.

Stage C: Invasion through the serosa, regional lymph node involvement.

Stage D: Distant metastases.

  E. Treatment.

      1. Surgery in all cases to avoid bowel obstruction for palliation or cure.

      2. Radiation therapy preoperatively and for recurrence.

      3. Chemotherapy (5-fluorouracil) for metastases, but it is of no proven efficacy.

      4. For solitary hepatic metastases (or confined to one lobe), resection results in a 20% to 40% 5-year survival rate.

DIARRHEA

  I. Definition.

Increased stool liquidity and weight (> 200 grams daily) frequently associated with stool frequency, urgency/incontinence, and perianal discomfort.

  II. Broad classification.

  A. Osmotic.

      1. Caused by poorly absorbed solute.

      2. Stops with fasting.

      3. *Osmotic gap >50.

  B. Secretory.

      1. Osmotic pressure same as plasma.

*Stool osmolarity measured $-[2(Na + K)]$.

  2. Watery, voluminous stools.

  3. Persists with fasting.

  4. No WBC, RBCs, or fat.

 C. Exudative/infectious.

  1. WBCs and RBCs in stool.

  2. Fever, chills.

  3. Leukocytosis.

  4. Culture positive.

III. Osmotic diarrhea.

 A. Differential diagnosis.

  1. Disaccharidase deficiency.

  2. Glucose-galactose/fructose malabsorption.

  3. Mannitol/sorbitol ingestion.

  4. Lactulose.

  5. Magnesium sulfate.

 B. Treatment.

  Avoidance and dietary restriction.

IV. Secretory diarrhea.

 A. Differential diagnosis.

  1. Toxigenic: cholera, *Escherichia coli.*

  2. Endocrine: Vasoactive intestinal peptide (VIP), calcitonin, prostaglandin, serotonin.

  3. Zollinger-Ellison: high gastrin levels.

  4. Villous adenoma: hypokalemia.

  5. Niacin deficiency: dermatitis and dementia.

  6. Collagen-vascular disease.

  7. Infections: tuberculosis, giardia, strongyloides.

V. Evaluation of diarrhea.

 A. Diagnosis proceeds based on a complete history. If the patient gives a history of an acute onset, one must first consider infectious causes, inflammatory bowel disease, *Clostridium difficile* pseudomembranous colitis, toxin induced, or perhaps fecal impaction. Evaluation should initially include:

  1. Stool examination for WBCs and RBCs, ova, and parasites and perhaps *C. difficile* toxin if the patient has previously taken antibiotics.

  2. If diarrhea persists, one may want to selectively pursue, some of the tests listed below. Tests

should be ordered on the basis of history. For example, if the patient provides a history suggestive of steatorrhea, one may want to test stool with a sudan stain (qualitative) and then if necessary supplement that with quantitative fat, D-xylose, and chymex tests.

3. Chronic causes of diarrhea imply different disorders such as cathartic abuse, endocrine disorders, lactase deficiency, malabsorption, lymphoma, and amyloid. Tests specific for these syndromes should be performed.

B. Proctoscopy.
   1. Yellowish plaques: seen in pseudomembranous colitis.
   2. Melanosis seen in laxative abuse.
   3. Adenoma.

C. Blood: complete blood cell (CBC) count, SMA-18, erythrocyte sedimentation rate (ESR), eosinophil count, thyroid function tests. May also need to measure cortisol, VIP calcitonin, gastrin, and prostaglandins.

D. X-ray (helpful in chronic syndromes): Upper GI study with small bowel and a barium enema study (for inflammatory bowel disease, lymphoma, sprue, etc.).

E. Small bowel studies.
   1. Aspirate: *Giardia*.
   2. Biopsy: Whipple's sprue.
   3. Mucosal disaccharidase studies.
   4. D-xylose: mucosal cause of malabsorption.
   5. CO_2-bile acid breath test: bile acid absorption.
   6. Chymex test: pancreatic malabsorption.

F. Colonoscopy with or without rectal biopsy.

G. Urine.
   1. 5-hydroxyindoleacetic acid (5-HIAA): carcinoid.
   2. Vanillylmandelic acid (VMA)/metanephrines: pheochromocytoma.
   3. Heavy metals: lead, arsenic, etc.

4. Alkalinization for phenolphthalein (laxative abuse).

VI. Treatment.

A. Monitor vital signs and orthostasis. Replace salt and water depletion with intravenous fluids (normal saline) if the clinical situation warrants.

B. Antibiotics for infectious causes.

C. For malabsorption, may give pancreatic enzymes.

D. Dietary manipulation: e.g., avoidance of milk products for lactose intolerance, removal of osmotic cause.

E. Therapy for specific causes: inflammatory bowel disease, endocrine causes.

F. Diphenoxylate hydrochloride with atropine sulfate (Lomotil): contraindicated in infectious causes.

VII. Infectious diarrhea (see Chapter 2).

INFLAMMATORY BOWEL DISEASE

I. General.

A. Crohn's disease (CD): a chronic inflammatory disease of the GI tract of unknown cause involving the entire length from mouth to anus. The inflammation is transmural with the distal ileum and colon most often affected. The peak incidence is between ages 15 to 30 years and is more common among Jews, people of European descent, and caucasians.

B. Ulcerative colitis (UC): an inflammatory disease of unknown cause involving most often only the mucosa of the colon beginning at the rectum and advancing proximally. Incidence rates reveal a bimodal distribution in the 3rd and 5th decades. The demographics for increased risk are similar to those of CD.

II. Pathologic findings.

A. CD: all layers of the bowel wall are thickened. Non-caseating granulomas are seen with an inflammatory process that is most intense in the submucosa with fissures and ulceration penetrating through the mucosal layer. The colon is involved in two thirds of the patients with the small bowel involved 80% of the time. The small bowel and colon are affected exclusively in patients 30% and 20% of the time, respectively.

B. UC: crypt abcesses are commonly seen but are not specific for this disease. Distorted crypt architecture, mixed lamina propria inflammation, crypt atrophy, basal lymphoid aggregates, and superficial erosions are seen more commonly in UC than in self-limited colitis.

III. Signs and symptoms.

A. CD: diarrhea, abdominal pain, anal/perirectal fissures and fistulae, and internal and cutaneous fistulae.

B. UC: diarrhea, hematochezia, fever, abdominal pain, anal and perirectal disease (less common than CD).

IV. Local complications.

A. CD: slightly increased risk for colon cancer, bleeding, abscess formation, fistulae, and bowel obstruction.

B. UC: massive colonic hemorrhage, colonic stricture, toxic megacolon, increased risk for colon cancer (especially when disease extends more proximally than sigmoid colon), and colonic perforation.

V. Systemic manifestations.

A. Arthritis: ankylosing spondylitis does not reflect disease activity, but peripheral arthritis appears to parallel disease activity.

B. Dermatologic: erythema nodosum and pyoderma gangrenosum (more common in UC) are occasionally present.

C. Hematologic: most often seen are anemia, thrombocytosis, and hypercoagulable states.

D. Hepatobiliary: cholelithiasis (cholesterol stones in CD), fatty liver (usually secondary to malnutrition, more common in CD), chronic active hepatitis, pericholangitis, sclerosing cholangitis (highly associated with UC), and cholangiocarcinoma.

  E. Renal: nephrolithiasis, ureteral obstruction (CD), and genitourinary tract-enteric fistulae (CD).

  F. Ophthalmologic: iritis and episcleritis are well-documented complications.

VI. Diagnosis.

  A. CD: colonoscopy with mucosal biopsy, and a small bowel barium study should be performed if disease excludes the colon.

  B. UC: colonscopy/sigmoidoscopy with mucosal biopsy or a barium enema study are recommended for initial evaluation.

VII. Therapy.

  A. Crohn's disease.

   1. Acute exacerbation:

    a. Sulfasalazine* 2.0–6.0 g/day.

    b. Prednisone 0.25–0.75 mg/kg/day.

    c. Metronidazole 800 mg/day.

    d. Azathioprine with steroids for steroid-sparing effect.

   2. Maintenance:

    a. Sulfasalazine in low doses is not significantly more effective than a placebo.

    b. Azathioprine (3.0 mg/kg/day) when given with steroids is more effective than a placebo.

  B. Ulcerative colitis.

   1. Acute exacerbation:

    a. Bowel rest with parenteral alimentation.

    b. Rectally administered steroids (e.g., corticosteroid enemas) in distal colitis.

    c. 5'Acetylsalicylic acid enemas in distal colitis.

    d. Parenteral antibiotics in severe colitis.

---

*Sulfasalazine should be started at 1 g/day and increased 500 mg to 1 g every 2 days pending tolerance of the drug until the desired dosage is obtained. Side effects include skin rash, platelet dysfunction, occasional bone marrow suppression, decreased sperm counts, interference with folate uptake, and precipitation of hemolysis in glucose-6-phosphate dehydrogenase-deficient patients.

2. Surgical indications:
   a. A total colectomy is indicated in cases in which aggressive medical management fails to control the acute disease process especially when hemorrhagic colitis, toxic megacolon, or perforation is present.
3. Maintenance:
   a. Sulfasalazine 2 g/day (500 mg four times a day).

MALABSORPTION

I. Definition.
   Impaired breakdown of food and/or uptake of nutrients in the GI tract. This can be categorized into three basic phases:
   A. Intraluminal phase: this can be further subdivided into digestion of protein and fat (e.g., pancreatic exocrine function), solubilization of fat (e.g., micellar formation), and availability of nutrients.
   B. Intestinal phase: includes brush border processes (e.g., carbohydrate breakdown) and normal mucosal function in transport of nutrients from the intestine into the epithelium.
   C. Lymphatic phase: transports fat and protein from epithelial cells to the lymphatics for systemic utilization.

II. Signs and symptoms.
   A. Diarrhea: 10% to 25% of patients may have steatorrhea without diarrhea.
   B. Weight loss: patients usually have normal or excessive caloric intake.
   C. Steatorrhea: bulky, pale, greasy stools with rancid odor.
   D. Increased flatulence/bloating.
   E. Abdominal pain and cramps.
   F. Anemia.
      1. Iron deficiency: usually associated with diffuse mucosal lesions of the proximal small bowel.

The patient may not have overt intestinal symptoms or steatorrhea as in some cases of celiac sprue.

2. Folate deficiency is associated with proximal small bowel disease.

3. Vitamin B12 deficiency is seen with bacterial overgrowth, terminal ileal disease, and surgical resection.

G. Eosinophilia is seen in eosinophilic gastroenteritis.

H. Bruising or bleeding tendencies may be indicative of vitamin K malabsorption.

I. Osteopenia is secondary to vitamin D and calcium malabsorption.

J. Muscle wasting.

K. Amenorrhea and infertility are associated with malnutrition.

L. Edema will be present in association with protein-losing enteropathies.

M. Glossitis.

III. Diagnostic tests.

There is a variety of tests described for the workup of malabsorption. Below are the most useful tests.

A. Tests for fat malabsorption.

1. A good qualitative test is the sudan stain, which is 80% to 90% sensitive. First, place a stool sample on a glass slide and homogenize with water or saline. Second, add a few drops of glacial acetic acid to hydrolyze the triglycerides and insoluble soaps of fatty acids to free fatty acids. Third, add sudan III stain in 70% alcohol and heat to boiling, and finally examine under the microscope while still warm. The size and number of fat droplets are increased in steatorrhea. Nonabsorbable fat (e.g., mineral oil or castor oil) will give false-positive results and inadequate fat intake can lead to false-negative results.

2. Fecal fat quantitation. First, place the patient on a 80–100 g fat diet for 2 days, and then col-

lect all stool while on the same diet for the next 3 days and keep refrigerated. Greater than 7–9 g of fecal fat excretion per day is indicative of fat malabsorption.

3. Carbon-14-triolein breath test is a radiolabeled triglyceride mixed with trioctanoin and cottonseed oil given to a fasting patient. Breath samples are collected at 3, 4, 5, and 6 hours and the amount of labeled carbon dioxide is measured. At least 3.5% of the dose of triolein is detected in normal patients and less than this is indicative of steatorrhea.

B. Evaluation of the small intestine.

1. D-xylose: this does not require intraluminal digestion to be absorbed; therefore it is a useful screening test for patients with diffuse mucosal disease. A 25-g oral dose of D-xylose is given and a 5 hour urine collection is obtained along with a 2 hour post serum level of D-xylose. Normal levels include at least 5 g of D-xylose in the urine and a serum level of at least 25 mg/dL. This test should be normal in patients with pancreatic insufficiency, hepatobiliary disease, or lymphatic obstruction. D-xylose absorption is decreased in most patients with mucosal malabsorption and bacterial overgrowth. False-positive results can occur in patients with delayed gastric emptying, renal insufficiency, ascites, or severe peripheral edema.

2. The lactose breath hydrogen test is used to detect lactase deficiency. After a basal measurement of hydrogen is made, the patient ingests a standard dose of lactose (1 g/kg) and subsequent measurements of hydrogen are made. An increase of greater than 20 ppm of hydrogen is indicative of lactose malabsorption (an early peak of hydrogen may also indicate bacterial overgrowth in the small bowel).

3. A small bowel barium study is relatively insen-

sitive and may be normal in patients with mild mucosal disease. This test may be helpful in differentiating intraluminal maldigestion from mucosal malabsorption.

4. A small bowel aspirate for bacteria with greater than 10 million colonies/mL is abnormal.

5. Bile acid breath test: Carbon-14-labeled bile acid is given orally and labeled carbon dioxide is measured in the breath. Bacterial deconjugation of the bile acids leads to increased exhaled labeled carbon dioxide. The test will also be abnormal in patients with extensive ileal disease or resection where absorption of bile salts is impaired.

6. Schilling's test: the absorption of labeled vitamin B12 should normalize after antibiotics when bacterial overgrowth is the cause. It will not normalize if there is extensive ileal disease or resection.

C. Evaluation of pancreatic exocrine function. Pancreatic insufficiency can lead to impairment of dietary fat absorption and in severe cases results in protein malabsorption. Although there are several tests to diagnose exocrine dysfunction, most are impractical.

1. Bentiromide-para-aminobenzoic acid (PABA) test: The main diagnostic usefulness of the test is that chymotrypsin is required to break down this compound to bentiromide and PABA. The PABA is then absorbed and excreted in the urine. The PABA level will be low in severe pancreatic insufficiency (enzyme output less than 5% of normal). False-low levels will occur in patients with decreased intestinal absorption, severe liver disease, diabetes, or renal disease.

2. Schilling's test: Labeled vitamin B12 absorption should normalize after pancreatic enzyme replacement if pancreatic insufficiency is the cause.

IV. Diseases of malabsorption (categorized by defective phase).

A. Intraluminal phase.

1. Chronic pancreatitis, cystic fibrosis, and pancreatic carcinoma are associated with inadequate enzyme and bicarbonate release.

2. Zollinger-Ellison syndrome is characterized by inactivation of pancreatic enzymes by excess acid secretion.

3. Postgastrectomy syndrome results in inadequate mixing of gastric contents with secreted enzymes.

4. Decreased bile salts are seen in chronic liver disease, biliary obstruction, ileal disease, and small intestine bacterial overgrowth.

5. Extensive small bowel resection causes fat and vitamin B12 malabsorption syndromes.

6. Decreased availability of nutrients.

   a. Pernicious anemia: decreased vitamin B12 due to low or absent intrinsic factor.

   b. Blind loop syndrome: decreased vitamin B12 due to bacterial utilization and uptake.

B. Intestinal phase.

1. Lactase deficiency (mucosal enzyme defect).

2. Conditions associated with extensive mucosal involvement.

   a. Crohn's disease.

   b. Celiac disease (sprue, gluten-sensitive enteropathy).

   c. Tropical sprue.

   d. Radiation enteritis.

   e. Eosinophilic gastroenteritis.

   f. Whipple's disease.

   g. Ischemia of small intestine.

   h. Extensive small bowel resection.

   i. Drugs (e.g., colchicine, neomycin).

3. Congenital transport abnormalities.

   a. Defective amino acid transport (e.g., Hartnup disease, cystinuria).

      b. Defective folate and vitamin B12 uptake.

      c. Abetalipoproteinemia: inability to form chylomicrons.

      d. Primary bile salt malabsorption.

  C. Lymphatic phase.

      1. Lymphangiectasia.

      2. Lymphoma.

      3. Carcinoid.

      4. Tuberculosis.

  D. Miscellaneous causes.

      1. Diabetes.

      2. Giardiasis.

      3. Adrenal insufficiency.

      4. Hyperthyroidism.

      5. Acquired immunodeficiency syndrome.

      6. Amyloidosis.

      7. Hypogammaglobulinemia.

ACUTE PANCREATITIS

  I. Signs and symptoms.
Epigastric pain boring through to back, vomiting, fever, distended abdomen with decreased bowel sounds, Cullen's sign (periumbilical blue discoloration), and Grey-Turner's sign (flank discoloration).

  II. Laboratory.
Elevated amylase and lipase. May also see elevated alkaline phosphatase and bilirubin, leukocytosis, hyperglycemia, and hypocalcemia.

  III. X-rays.

      1. Kidneys, ureters, bladder: Sentinel loop (air-filled small bowel), nonspecific ileus.

      2. Ultrasound (US) or computed tomography (CT): Diffusely enlarged pancreas. May also see a pseudocyst.

  IV. Etiology.
Ethanol, cholelithiasis, idiopathic, drugs (e.g., furosemide, steroids, thiazides, azathioprine), hyperlipidemia, trauma.

V. Ranson's criteria (predicts morbidity and mortality).
Poor prognosis associated with:
  1. WBC count > 15,000/mm^3.
  2. Glucose > 150 mg/dL. With no history of hyperglycemia.
  3. Albumin < 3.2 g/dL.
  4. BUN > 45 mg/dL.
  5. PaO$_2$ < 60 mm Hg.
  6. Serum calcium < 8.0 mg/dL.
  7. LDH > 600 U/dL.
  8. SGOT and SGPT > 200 U/dL.
  9. Base deficit > 4 mEq/L.
  10. Fluid sequestration > 6 L.
  11. Hematocrit decrease > 10%.

VI. Mortality related to Ransom's criteria.

No. of risk factors	Mortality
0–2	<10%
3–4	25%–30%
5–6	50%
7–8	95%

VII. Treatment (generally supportive and symptomatic).
  1. The patient should have nothing to eat or drink. Nasogastric suction should only be used for persistent vomiting.
  2. Intravenous hydration should be used to replace sequestered fluids and to maintain normal volume status.
  3. Meperidine is used for pain because it has little effect on the sphincter of Oddi.
  4. If the patient remains febrile, abdominal US is indicated to exclude gallstones, biliary stricture (or tumor), as well as pancreatic pseudocyst or abscess. Abdominal CT may have a higher diagnostic yield for abscess or pseudocyst.

HEPATITIS

A. Various Hepatitis B (HBV) serologic markers.

   1. HBcAg: Core antigen from viral nucleocapsid. Not commonly seen in the circulation and obtained with a liver biopsy specimen.

   2. Anti-HBc: Antibody to HBcAg. Good screen for HBV infection past and present, carrier and noncarrier. Measures IgG level.

   3. Anti-HBc IgM: Elevated in acute infection and can remain at low levels for months after recovery. Uses: to identify other causes of liver damage in healthy carriers, and to prove recent acute HBV infection if HBsAb is negative.

   4. HBeAg: Thought to be excess HBcAg that is released into the serum as a smaller molecule. This antigen is associated with active replication and therefore increased infectivity.

   5. Anti-HBe: Usually signifies decreased infectivity although some patients may still be infectious.

   6. Delta virus (HDAg): When present in the serum, it indicates an acute infection. Since it peaks early in the infection, sensitivity is low and a negative HDAg does not rule out an acute delta infection.

   7. Anti-HD: This includes antiHD-IgM and antiHD-IgG. Although more specific antibodies are used experimentally, they are not commercially available. This is elevated in acute and chronic HDV infection; however, Anti-HD IgG is the predominant immunoglobulin in chronic infections.

B. Hepatitis A (HAV) serology.

   1. Anti-HAV IgM: Present in acute HAV infection. Peaks within 3 weeks and can persist at low levels for up to several months.

   2. Anti-HAV IgG: Not present in the acute infection. Peaks between 3 to 12 months after the onset of illness.

C. Tests for acute Viral Hepatitis.
1. Anti-HAV IgM.
2. Anti-HB core IgM.
3. HBs antigen.

Viral hepatitis can be characterized by its incubation period, serology, and high risk groups. Signs and symptoms may overlap. Table 5–1 demonstrates these characteristics and includes the course of the illness, treatment, and prophylaxis.

FULMINANT HEPATIC FAILURE

I. Definition.
Occurs in an injured liver when the balance between hepatic necrosis and regeneration is threatened leading to metabolic and neuropsychiatric changes.

II. Causes.
Viral (Hepatitis A; B; non-A, non-B; delta agent), drugs (isoniazid, tylenol, halothane), toxins, metabolic (Wilson's disease, fatty liver of pregnancy), vascular (Budd-Chiari syndrome, cardiogenic shock), immunocompromised (herpes simplex, cytomegalovirus).

III. Physical examination.
A. Neurologic.
1. Focal neurologic deficits may be secondary to intracranial hemorrhage from associated coagulopathy.
2. Four stages of hepatic coma.
Stage I: Slow response to questions with or without asterixis.
Stage II: Drowsy, responds to simple commands plus asterixis.
Stage III: Stuporous, responsive to pain.
Stage IV: Unresponsive to pain.
B. General Physical Examination. Decreased liver span, ascites, collateral vessels.

IV. Laboratory assessment.
A. SGOT/SGPT: Marked elevation; low enzymes may indicate no liver reserve.

TABLE 5–1.
Hepatitis

	Type				
Description	A	B	Non A Non B	Delta	
Virus	27 nm ss RNA	42 nm ds DNA	Not isolated	35-37 nm	
Incubation	2-6 wk	4-24 wk	1-12 wk	4-35 wk	
Transmission	Fecal-oral	Parenteral, sexual, maternal-fetal	Parenteral; most common hepatitis with blood transfusion	Parenteral, can be a co-infection or super infection with HBV	
High-risk groups	Homosexuals, institutionalized, day care exposure, shellfish ingestion	Homosexuals, intravenous drug users, institutionalized, hemodialysis, relatives	Institutionalized, blood recipients	Same as HBV, especially hemophiliacs and intravenous drug abusers	
History	Nausea, anorexia, low grade fever, light stools, dark urine, tender right upper quadrant, jaundice (Note: may be subclinical)	Similar to hepatitis A, fever less common, often more insidious onset, may also be subclinical	Often fewer symptoms than others	Superinfection of HDV can occur in HBsAg carriers and will cause a transient hepatitis and is usually more severe than when the patient has an acute HBV infection alone	

Diagnosis	IgM antibody to hepatitis A; transaminases 10 times normal	Hepatitis B surface antigen, hepatitis B anti-core	No specific marker; diagnosis of exclusion	Anti-HDV associated with HBsAg (+), anti-HBc-Igm (+) for acute co-infection or with HBsAg (+), anti-HBc-IgM (−) for superinfections in the chronic carrier of HBV
Course	Rarely fatal, no chronic carriers, no cirrhosis	Fatal 1%, 5%-10% chronic carriers, can lead to cirrhosis, increased hepatoma risk	Can be fatal, can be chronic, can lead to cirrhosis	Coinfections are usually more severe and have a higher incidence of fulminant hepatitis than HBV alone. Chronic HDV infections can be more aggressive than HBV alone
Treatment	Symptomatic; hospitalize if: severely dehydrated, there is a prolongation in the prothrombin time, or marked bilirubin elevation. Assure adequate fluids, restrict protein, avoid sedation, avoid acetaminophen, and follow up prothrombin time. Check ammonia level and give lactulose if encephalopathy develops.			
Prophylaxis	Serum immune globulin, .02-1 mL/kg post exposure and if traveling to endemic area	Hepatitis B immune globulin: for spouses, needle exposure, infants of infected mothers, vaccine for high risk	None	None, however, HBV immunization will prevent co- and superinfection

   B. LDH: Sensitive indicator of ongoing necrosis because of a short half-life.

   C. Arterial blood gas: Respiratory alkalosis, metabolic acidosis.

   D. Coagulation factors: Diminished except factor VIII.

   E. Fibrinogen and fibrin split products: May detect disseminated intravascular coagulation (DIC).

   F. Ammonia: Correlates poorly with encephalopathy.

   G. PaO_2: 30% develop adult respiratory distress syndrome.

   H. Glucose: Decreased secondary to loss of gluconeogenesis.

V. Management.

   A. Supportive care to allow time for hepatic regeneration. Therapy is directed by the level of hepatic coma. Major causes of death are cerebral edema and hemorrhage, sepsis, and renal failure.

   B. Therapy.

      1. Lactulose 30 mL by mouth three times a day (or per nasogastric tube or 100–200 g/200 mL H_2O as an enema) titrated to two to three stools per day is given to reduce encephalopathy. Neomycin (6–8 g/day) in divided doses has been given as an alternative to lactulose but has renal and ototoxicity.

      2. Glucose given intravenously with frequent monitoring of blood sugar to avoid hypoglycemia.

      3. Vitamin K/FFP should be given to maintain factors II, V, VII, and X at levels greater than 50% to avoid hemorrhage. If factor VIII (synthesized in the capillary wall, *not* the liver) is low, DIC may be present and cryoprecipitate should be considered.

      4. Histamine-blockers should be used prophylactically to prevent stress ulcerations.

      5. Antibiotics should be used if sepsis is suspected. Likely sources include peritonitis, meningitis, urinary tract infections, and infections of intravenous lines. Common organisms in-

clude *Escherichia coli*, staphylococci, and streptococci.

6. Liver transplantation in the appropriate patient should be considered.

7. Avoid sedatives since many are hepatically metabolized and will prevent adequate assessment of mental status.

8. For stages III and IV coma, mannitol should be given (1 g/kg intravenously) to reduce cerebral edema. This is done only if serum osmolarity is less than 320.

9. Careful attention must be paid to electrolytes, hemoglobin, and platelet levels.

10. If acetaminophen overdose is suspected, N-acetyl-cysteine is used within the first 16 hours of ingestion. Once fulminant hepatic failure begins there is no use for this agent.

CIRRHOSIS

I. Definition.
   Cirrhosis is a condition of fibrosis and nodular regeneration following hepatocellular necrosis and may result from a number of different causes.

II. Causes.
   A. Viral: Hepatitis B, Non-A, Non-B.
   B. Metabolic: Wilson's disease, alpha-1-antitrypsin deficiency, hemochromatosis.
   C. Cholestasis: primary biliary cirrhosis (PBC), primary sclerosing cholangitis, autoimmune chronic active hepatitis.
   D. Toxin/drugs: methotrexate, isoniazid, amiodarone.
   E. Cryptogenic.

III. Lab tests.
   A. Biochemistry levels: Alkaline phosphatase, serum leucine aminopeptidase, and 5-nucleotidase are markers for cholestasis. Serum protein electrophoresis may reveal an elevated polydispersed gamma-globulin fraction. Albumin is a marker of protein

synthesis but may also be low in patients with malnutrition and protein-losing enteropathies. Cholesterol is also a marker of hepatic function and can be elevated in cholestasis (vide supra).

B. Prothrombin time: Can be prolonged because of poor hepatic function or vitamin K deficiency. A coagulation profile drawn before the administration of vitamin K can differentiate these causes. Factors II, V, VII, IX, and X are all produced in the liver; however, factor V is not a vitamin K dependent factor and should be normal in a vitamin K deficient patient. Factor V may be abnormal in liver disease or disseminated intravascular coagulation (DIC). A normal factor VIII level which is produced primarily outside the liver will be low in DIC but normal or elevated in liver disease.

C. Specific tests:

1. Alpha-1-antitrypsin level and phenotype.
2. 24-hour urine sample for copper levels, and serum ceruloplasmin for Wilson's disease.
3. Iron, total iron binding capacity, and ferritin level for hemochromatosis.
4. Anti-mitochondrial antibodies for primary biliary cirrhosis.
5. Anti-smooth muscle antibodies and anti-nuclear antibody for autoimmune chronic active hepatitis.
6. Alpha-fetoprotein for hepatoma.

IV. A liver biopsy specimen provides the most information as to the state and possible cause of the liver disease.

A. Percutaneous biopsy is the quickest and safest route. It is contraindicated when ascites is present or if there is an active right lower lung process. It is also contraindicated in the presence of a severe coagulopathy, or in an uncooperative patient. Complications include hemorrhage and pneumothorax.

B. Open liver biopsy is relatively safe and can be performed in cases of a coagulopathy. A transvenous biopsy can be performed with coagulopathy but the specimen size is usually very small.

V. CT and US of the abdomen can facilitate assessment of the parenchyma and demonstrate mass lesions (i.e., hepatoma).

VI. Endoscopy of the upper GI tract is not standard in the evaluation of liver disease; however, if the patient is anemic and the stools are positive for blood, it would be indicated. Approximately 50% to 60% of upper GI bleeding in cirrhosis is due to esophageal varices.

VII Treatment needs to be tailored to the individual. The following are just guidelines and are not meant to be all inclusive:

   A. Remove offending agent (e.g., drugs, alcohol, etc.).
   B. Nutritional support.
   C. Phlebotomy for hemochromatosis.
   D. Steroids for autoimmune hepatitis.
   E. D-penicillamine administration in cases of Wilson's disease.
   F. Colchicine and methotrexate may be of benefit in the appropriate patient (i.e., alcoholic cirrhosis and primary biliary cirrhosis, respectively); however, they are still in the investigational stage.
   G. Orthotopic liver transplantation is an option in patients with end-stage liver disease, but the indications and eligibility for this are complex and beyond the scope of this section.

VIII. Complications of cirrhosis and treatment.

   A. Ascites and portal hypertension: Clinically these patients are frequently volume overloaded although their effective circulation is low. They should be sodium (2 g/day) and fluid restricted. If massive ascites is present and compromises patient activity or respiratory function, paracentesis should be performed. An ascites sample drawn for diagnostic purposes should be sent for culture, cell count, cytologic studies, pH, albumin, amylase, and LDH levels. A WBC count of greater than 300 polymorphonuclear leukocytes is seen in bacterial peritonitis and should be treated with appropriate antibiotic therapy. If the ascites is intractable, a LeVeen shunt can be placed. Complications associated with these shunts include DIC, infection, and congestive heart failure due to the sudden increase in intravascular volume.

B. Encephalopathy.

1. Lactulose: 30 mL by mouth titrated to elicit two to three stools per day. If the patient is too lethargic, this can be given as an enema (300 mL lactulose with 700 ml water).

2. Protein restriction.

3. Neomycin: 0.5 g every 6 hours if the patient is not already on parenteral antibiotics or lactulose.

C. Variceal hemorrhage (see GI bleeding).

1. Sclerotherapy can be an effective treatment for variceal bleeding.

2. A portacaval shunt can be placed, but has a higher incidence of encephalopathy.

Due to the poor underlying condition of most of these patients, the mortality rate associated with variceal bleeding remains high.

BIBLIOGRAPHY

Gastroenterology and Hepatology

Ahtone M: Hepatitis B diagnosis. *JAMA* 1983; 249:2068.

Geokas MC, et al: Acute pancreatitis. *Ann Intern Med* 1985; 103:86–100.

Jensen DM; Portal-systemic encephalopathy and hepatic coma. *Med Clin N Am* 1986; 70:108–1092.

Marzuk PM, Schwartz JS; Endoscopic sclerotherapy for esophageal varices. *Ann Intern Med* 1984; 100:608–610.

Payne JA: Fulminant liver failure. *Med Clin N Am* 1986; 70:1067–1079.

Ranson JHC: Etiological and prognostic factors in human acute pancreatitis: A review. *Am J Gastroenterol* 1982; 77:633–638.

Schaffner J: Gastrointestinal bleeding. *Med Clin N Am* 1986; 70:1055–1066.

Sherlock S: *Diseases of the Liver and Biliary System*, ed 7. Oxford, Blackwell Scientific Publications, 1985.

Sleisenger MH, Fordtran JS: *Gastrointestinal Diseases*, ed 3. Philadelphia, WB Saunders Co, 1983.

Winawer SJ, Sherlock P: Surveillance for colorectal cancer in average-risk groups, familial high-risk groups, and patients with adenomas. *Cancer* 1982; 50:2609–2614.

Hematology

Pat Murphy, M.D.
Ed Priest, M.D.
Larry Cripe, M.D.

HEMOSTASIS AND DISORDERS OF HEMOSTASIS

I. Introduction.

A. Normal hemostasis.

Definition: cessation of bleeding from an injured vessel requires a complex interaction between blood vessels, platelets, and the coagulation proteins.

After blood vessel injury, the smooth muscle constricts and platelets adhere to vessel walls creating an initial plug. This action along with further platelet recruitment and aggregation is referred to as primary hemostasis. Primary hemostasis (platelet function and number) is adequately tested with bleeding time. Clinically, platelet defects may be suggested by petechiae or mucous membrane oozing.

Secondary hemostasis refers to the complex sequence of events resulting in retraction and stabilization of the platelet plug. A series of activated coagulation proteins convert prothrombin to thrombin (Fig 6–1). Thrombin is an important mediator of further vessel constriction, platelet aggregation, and conversion of fibrinogen to fibrin. Defects in the coagulation cascade may be suggested by large ecchymosis, hemarthrosis, or extensive bleeding from trauma.

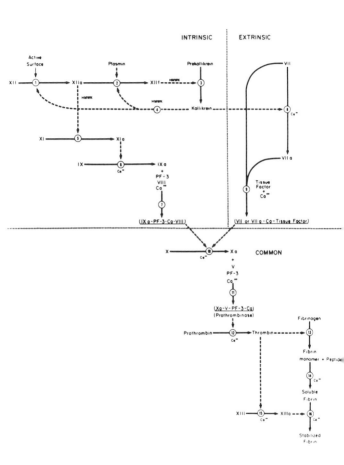

FIG 6–1

The interactions of the coagulation factors. A modification of the cascade or waterfall hypothesis of McFarlane and of Davie and Ratnoff. The three pathways of coagulation are separated by *dotted lines.* A *solid arrow* indicates transformation; a *dashed arrow* denotes action. Complex enzymes are *underlined* and enclosed in parenthesis; e.g., (Xa-V-PF-3-Ca). *PF-3* = platelet factor 3; *HMWK* = high molecular weight kininogen. (From Wintrobe MM: *Clinical Hematology,* ed 8. Philadelphia, Lea & Febiger, 1981. Used by permission.)

B. Routine laboratory evaluation.
   1. Peripheral smear: special aspects will be discussed throughout this section.
   2. Platelet count: the normal platelet count is between 150,000–450,000 platelets/mm^3.
   3. Prothrombin time (PT): this test facilitates evaluation of the extrinsic and common pathways (Fig 6–1). Factors II, V, VII, and X are assessed. The PT reflects the synthetic capacity of the liver, vitamin K availability, and alterations of coumarin therapy. The PT should be followed up when the coumarin level is adjusted.
   4. Activated partial thromboplastin time (PTT): this test facilitates evaluation of the intrinsic and common pathways (Fig 6–1). Factors V, VIII, IX, X, XI, XII are assessed. The PTT will be altered by heparin therapy.
C. Other pertinent laboratory tests.
   1. Bleeding time: a reliable index of platelet function.
   2. Thrombin time (TT): facilitates assessment of the coagulation cascade distal to the formation of thrombin (Fig 6–1). The TT may be abnormal in the presence of heparin, fibrinogen defects, or problems with fibrin polimerization.
   3. Other useful studies might include fibrinogen concentration, fibrin split products, individual coagulation protein assays, and von Willebrand activity.

II. Platelet disorders.
A. Thrombocytopenia (platelet count <150,000/mm^3).
   1. Thrombocytopenia may result from three primary mechanisms: decreased or ineffective production, decreased survival, or sequestration in the spleen.

Note: False-positive results in both the PT and the PTT may occur with inadequate volume sampling and sampling from a heparin-containing catheter.

Decreased or ineffective production of platelets may be the result of primary bone marrow failure (e.g., aplastic anemia), a myelophthistic process (tumor or infection replacing the marrow), selective drug toxicity (alcohol, anticonvulsants, thiazides, and insecticides), or megaloblastic processes (folic acid or vitamin B12 deficiency).

The peripheral smear may give you a clue to the mechanism of thrombocytopenia. Young platelets are large and clump easily. A preponderance of these may suggest a destructive process while small, older platelets may suggest ineffective production. Severe macrocytosis may suggest a nutritional deficiency although both aplastic anemia and myelodysplastic syndromes may cause mild macrocytosis. Nucleated RBCs and teardrop RBCs may suggest a myelophthistic process or sequestration, while fragmented RBCs should alert you to the possible diagnosis of thrombotic thrombocytopenia purpura (TTP) or the hemolytic-uremic syndrome.

2. Specific causes.
   a. Immune thrombocytopenia. Immune thrombocytopenia without a clear cause (infection, post transfusion, drugs including quinine, quinidine, sulfonamide derivatives, or collagen vascular disease) is referred to as idiopathic thrombocytopenia purpura (ITP). Acute ITP mainly affects children. Therapy is not necessary unless mucous membrane bleeding occurs. Some physicians treat all adults with Prednisone 1–2 mg/kg/day initially. Chronic ITP is more common in women and men who are homosexuals. The diagnosis should be suspect if splenomegaly is present. This disease is characterized by remissions and relapses,

which make therapeutic guidelines difficult. If steroid therapy fails or an unacceptable steroid dose is required to maintain a platelet count greater than 50,000/mm^3, splenectomy may be necessary.

b. Thrombotic thrombocytopenia purpura. TTP is an acute medical emergency characterized by microangiopathic hemolytic anemia, thrombocytopenia, fluctuating neurologic changes, azotemia, and fever. TTP is rare and frequently fatal. Plasma infusions and/or plasmaphoresis are the treatment of choice, although this continues to be controversial. Platelet transfusions should be avoided.

c. Disseminated intravascular coagulation (DIC). This is a syndrome of multiple causes characterized by fibrin formation in the microcirculation and the development of fibrinolysis. Hemorrhagic complications are more common than thrombotic problems. DIC is always secondary to another disorder including obstetric complications, malignancies, liver disease, extensive burns, or infections. There is no specific laboratory diagnosis. Abnormalities include thrombocytopenia, prolonged PT and PTT, and possible RBC fragments on peripheral smears. Fibrinogen levels are usually decreased. Factor VIII is also decreased, which suggests a process more extensive than vitamin K or liver disease since this factor is produced by endothelial cells.

Treatment should be aimed at the underlying disorders. In patients with significant bleeding, fresh frozen plasma may be used (2–10 U/day). Cryoprecipitate, which contains high concentrations of fibrinogen, may be used to elevate fibrinogen levels to greater than 100 mg/dL. Platelets may be useful. Heparin therapy continues to be controversial and should only be used as a last resort and with expert guidance.

3. Platelet transfusions.

Bleeding complications secondary to thrombocytopenia rarely occur with platelet counts greater than 60,000/mm³. Platelet counts between 40,000/mm³ and 60,000/mm³ may be associated with bleeding following trauma or surgical procedures. A platelet count greater than 50,000/mm³ may be adequate for lumbar puncture. Spontaneous bleeding may occur with platelet counts less than 20,000/mm³.

Platelet transfusions are useful in patients with severe thrombocytopenia secondary to ineffective production. As a general rule, patients with thrombocytopenia secondary to destructive/sequestration processes will not respond to transfusions. Platelet transfusions in these patients should be reserved for bleeding complications.

Random donor platelets comprise platelets from six volunteers. These are the initial mainstay of transfusions. Random platelet packs present a variety of antigens to the host. In patients requiring multiple platelet transfusions (treatment of leukemia, bone marrow transplantation), less antigenic platelets may be required as the host becomes sensitized to the transfusions. This may include single-donor platelets or HLA identical platelets.

B. Thrombocytosis (platelet count >400,000/mm³). Thrombocytosis is rarely associated with thrombotic or hemorrhagic complications and is almost always associated with platelet counts greater than 400,000/mm³. Secondary or reactive thrombocytosis is associated with hemorrhage, hemolysis, infections, inflammatory diseases, carcinoma, and lymphomas. These are rarely associated with platelet counts greater than 1 million.

Primary or essential thrombocythemia is usually encountered in myeloproliferative disorders. Many features are similar to polycythemia rubra vera but in essential thrombocythemia a low or normal hemoglobin level should be present. Splenomegaly is present in 40% to 80%.

C. Qualitative platelet disorders. These are associated with an abnormal bleeding time despite a normal platelet count. These defects are most commonly associated with acquired disorders, particularly drugs. Non-steroidal antiinflammatory drugs inhibit platelet function. Other important drugs include aminophylline, heparin, ethanol, and penicillins, especially carbenicillin. Other causes include uremia, paraproteinemias, and hepatic cirrhosis.

Except for von Willebrand's disease, congenital qualitative platelet defects are rare. These include Bernard-Soulier syndrome and thrombosthenia.

III. Coagulation disorders.

A. Diseases manifested by an abnormal PTT (normal PT, thrombin time, and platelet count).

1. Spurious: Prolongation may occur with an inadequate volume sample or drawing blood from heparin-containing catheters.

2. Factor VIII or IX deficiency (hemophilia A or B, respectively): Hemophilia A is the most common congenital disorder of blood coagulation. Hemophilia A and B occur as sex-linked recessive diseases and thus occur in men. The disease usually manifests itself at an early age and is characterized by bleeding in the joints, especially in knees, elbows and ankles. This results in severe pain and swelling, and may eventually lead to deformity and crippling. Extensive bleeding may also occur in soft tissue and muscles.

Diagnosis is suggested by the bleeding pattern and family history. The definitive diagnosis is made with findings of a factor VIII activity assay.

Treatment is usually the administration of factor VIII during bleeding episodes. The fundamentals of replacement therapy for factor VIII deficiency may be generalized to other coagulation factor deficiencies. Normal plasma is assumed to contain 1 unit of factor VIII activity per milliliter. Bleeding complications do not occur if at least 50% of this activity is maintained. Patients with mild hemophilia (5% to 25% activity) may have significant bleeding with trauma or surgery. Severe, spontaneous hemorrhage usually does not occur unless the activity is less than 5% and many times less than 1%.

Early hemarthroses may be managed by maintaining plasma activity of factor VIII at 25% to 50% of normal for 2 to 3 days. Other significant hemorrhage may require a more prolonged treatment and maintaining a higher activity level (40% to 50% of normal). Prior to major surgery, patients should have 70% activity.

As mentioned, each milliliter of normal plasma contains 1 unit of factor VIII activity, thus fresh frozen plasma contains the equivalent amount. Cryoprecipitate contains approximately 100 units of factor VIII per milliliter and commercially prepared concentrates of factor VIII show the activity on the label. Factor VIII has a half-life of 10 to 12 hours and should be given twice a day. Knowing the units of each form of factor VIII and that the plasma volume is 40 mL/kg, the amount of factor VIII needed can be determined to maintain a specific activity.

3. Von Willebrand's disease.
   This is an autosomal dominant disease charac-

terized by an abnormal PTT, a prolonged
bleeding time (may be normal in 25% of patients), and abnormal platelet aggregation in response to the antibiotic ristocetin. The clinical
spectrum ranges from no symptoms to severe,
spontaneous bleeding. For most, the disease is
usually mild and becomes troublesome only
with trauma, surgery, or dental extractions.
Gastrointestinal hemorrhage is common.

4. Factor XI deficiency.
   This is an unusual disease usually affecting
   people of Jewish or Japanese descent. The
   hemorrhagic diathesis is mild with bleeding occurring after surgical or dental procedures.
   Plasma infusion usually controls hemorrhage.

5. Factor XII, prekallekrein, or high-molecular-
   weight kininogen deficiency.
   These disorders present with a prolonged PTT
   but do not have clinical manifestations.

6. Heparin therapy.

7. Circulating anticoagulants.
   Acquired inhibitors of coagulation factors may
   develop. These are especially seen in hemophil-
   iac patients who have received multiple transfusions. An antibody directed against
   phospholipid has been identified in patients
   with systemic lupus erythematosus (SLE).
   There is usually prolongation of both PTT and
   occasionally PT. These patients usually have no
   ill effects, though paradoxically thrombosis is
   more common than anticoagulation.

   Acquired inhibitors may also be associated
   with the postpartum period and rarely with
   drugs.

B. Diseases manifested by an abnormal PT (normal or
   elevated PTT, normal thrombin time, and normal
   bleeding time).

   Most commonly an isolated elevation of the PT
   is the result of warfarin therapy, liver disease, or vi-

tamin K deficiency. In the liver, vitamin K acts as an important cofactor in the posttranslational production of factors II (prothrombin), VII, IX, and X. The PT is very sensitive to alterations in factor VII. Severe vitamin K deficiency or profound liver disease may also prolong the PTT as a result of disruption of the common pathway.

C. Disease manifested by an abnormal PT, PTT, and thrombin time.

Disruption of all pathways may occur with severe liver disease, high dose heparin, DIC, or dysfibrinogenemia.

NEUTROPHILIC DISORDERS

I. Qualitative disorders.

Neutrophils are essential components of the immune system. Their primary function of killing microorganisms require that the cells: find the microorganism (chemotaxis), ingest the microorganism, and destroy the microorganism. Dysfunction may occur at any of these steps. Congenital disorders of neutrophils including Chediak-Higashi disease and others are beyond the scope of this text. It is important to remember that systemic diseases (diabetes, uremia, cirrhosis, burns) and drugs (corticosteroids) may alter neutrophil function.

II. Quantitative disorders.

A. Neutropenia.

Neutropenia is defined as an absolute neutrophil count of less than 1,500 neutrophils/mm³. A neutrophil count of less than 500 neutrophils/mm³ greatly increases the risk of serious infection. The etiology of neutropenia may be defined by whether the major mechanism is related to decreased bone marrow production or increased peripheral destruction.

1. Decreased bone marrow proliferation.

Severe neutropenia most commonly is the result of a drug-induced, dose-related hypoproliferation secondary to oncologic chemotherapeutic agents. Patients being treated with aggressive chemotherapeutic regimens; i.e., leukemia, lymphoma or bone marrow transplant patients, should have their neutrophil counts monitored daily. Signs and symptoms of infection must be treated with broad-spectrum antibiotics when neutrophil counts decrease to less than 500 neutrophils/mm^3.

Other drugs that may cause a dose-related neutropenia include chloramphenicol, ethanol, chlorpromazine, imipramine, and others. Some drugs may cause an idiosyncratic or hypersensitivity reaction unrelated to dose and rarely result in agranulocytosis. These include chloramphenicol, phenothiazines, phenylbutazone, sulfonamides, quinidine, procainamide, and penicillin.

Aplastic anemia, marrow infiltration (myelophthiasis), myelodysplastic syndromes, and megaloblastic anemia are important causative factors in patients with neutropenia. A bone marrow aspirate is required for definitive diagnosis, but the peripheral smear may give important clues. Marked macrocytosis and hypersegmentation of neutrophils suggest megaloblastic anemia although mild macrocytosis is common in aplastic anemia and myelodysplastic syndromes. Marrow infiltration is suggested by a leukoerythroblastic picture (i.e., a marked left shift with myelocytes, nucleated red blood cells, large platelets, and fragmented RBCs).

2. Increased peripheral destruction or sequestration.

   Destruction of neutrophils may occur in an autoimmune process such as in SLE or Felty's syndrome. Sequestration may occur in patients with hypersplenism.

B. Neutrophilia.

   Introduction: Neutrophilia is defined as an absolute neutrophil count greater than 10,000 cells/mm³. Most neutrophilia is associated with acute stress, acute and chronic inflammation, infection, tumors, or drugs (e.g., steroids). This neutrophilia may represent an increased marrow proliferation and demargination of WBCs into the bloodstream. The neutrophilia is usually mild-to-moderate (10,000–25,000 cells/mm³) with increased early forms (left shift). Neutrophilia between 50,000–100,000 cells/mm³ or rarely greater than 100,000 cells/mm³ with an elevated leukocyte alkaline phosphotase level represent a leukemoid reaction. A leukemoid reaction may occur in response to persistent infection (osteomyelitis, emphysema, septicemia, or tuberculosis), carcinoma (lung, stomach, breast, or liver), or Hodgkin's disease.

This response may be difficult to differentiate from chronic myelogenous leukemia. Chronic granulomatous leukemia should be considered when: the WBC count is greater than 100,000; there are many very early forms (including blast cells); increased numbers of basophils and eosinophils, and when splenomegaly is present.

C. Abnormal cells on a peripheral smear.

An absolute increase in the cells of a particular subclass (eosinophils, basophils, or monocytes) occur in a variety of diseases.

Lymphocytosis can be occasionally differentiated with peripheral smears. Atypical mature lymphocytes usually suggest a benign etiology, including infectious mononucleosis, viral hepatitis, allergic reaction, or other viral illnesses. Normal lymphocytes may suggest acute infections but may reveal chronic lymphocytic leukemia.

Bizarre, immature cells should alert you to the diagnosis of acute leukemia. A complete discussion of the leukemias and lymphomas is beyond the scope of this text.

TABLE 6–1.
Normal Blood Cell and Coagulation Values*

Parameter	Men	Women
WBC count (mL₃)†	7.25 (3.9–10.6)	7.28 (3.5–11.0)
RBC count (10^6/μL)†	5.11 (4.4–5.9)	4.51 (3.8–5.2)
Hemaglobin (g/dl)†	15.5 (13.3–17.7)	13.7 (11.7–15.7)
Hematocrit (5)†	46.0 (39.8–52.2)	40.9 (34.9–46.9)
MCV (um₃)†	90.1 (80.5–99.7)	90.4 (80.0–100.0)
aPTTT	21–31 sec	
PT	11–14 sec	
Procoagulant factors		
Fibrinogen	200–400 mg%	
Factors II, V, VII, X	70%–130%	
VIIIc	50%–200%	
Bleeding time	3–9 min	

*Adapted from Williams WJ et al: *Textbook of Hematology*, ed 3. New York,
McGraw Hill Book Co, 1983.
†Mean and range (mean ± 2 standard deviation). The mean represents the
normal white population. The range for blacks is 1 g/dL lower for men and
women.

ANEMIA

I. Anemia: General concepts.

Definition: A decrease in RBC mass generally reflected by the hemoglobin or the hematocrit level.

A. Signs and symptoms.

All patients suspected of having anemia should be
questioned and examined closely for evidence of
blood loss, nutritional deficiencies, toxin exposure
(ethanol especially), and a family history of anemia.
General signs and symptoms of anemia include:
weakness, fatigue, palpitations, dyspnea, dizziness,
headache, pallor, tachycardia, and systolic flow
murmurs.

B. Laboratory.

All patients being evaluated for anemia should have
a complete blood count including RBC indices, a
differential leukocyte count, and a platelet count
(Table 6–1).

1. Hemoglobin (Hg) and hematocrit (Hct) are estimates of the RBC mass. These values reflect the concentration of RBCs (Hct) or hemoglobin (Hg) within the circulation. Changes in the plasma volume, such as congestive heart failure or dehydration, may falsely decrease or increase these values respectively. Likewise, acute bleeding with rapid loss of blood may represent an anemia not reflected by the Hg or Hct.

2. Mean cell volume represents an average of the cell volume. This is one of the most important characteristics of an anemia and should be known in all cases. Early red cells (reticulocytes) are larger than more mature cells and a large percentage of early cells (as seen with brisk hemolysis for example) may raise the MCV.

3. Peripheral blood smear should be examined in all suspected cases of anemia and should assess:

   a. Anisocytosis: an abnormal variation in the size of red cells. This is reflected by an elevated red cell distribution width (RDW). Normal RBC size approximates that of the nucleus of a small lymphocyte (approximately 7 μ in diameter).

   b. Poikilocytosis: an abnormal variation in the shape of red cells. This includes elliptocytes, spherocytes, sickled cells, target cells, teardrop cells, and schistocytes.

   c. Polychromasia: a bluish tinge in young, large red cells. With supravital stains, these represent reticulocytes.

   d. Howell-Jolly bodies: remnants of nuclear material suggesting asplenia and may be present in severe anemias.

4. Reticulocyte count reflects the adequacy of the bone marrow in response to an anemia and can

help differentiate anemia caused by bone marrow failure from that associated with accelerated destruction or loss. From the reticulocyte count and the Hct, the reticulocyte production index (RPI) can be calculated.

This represents a measure of effective erythropoiesis for the degree of anemia.

$$RPI = \frac{\text{Reticulocyte count (\%)} \times \text{Hct}}{\text{Maturation factor* } \times \ (0.45)}$$

*Maturation factor

Hct	Maturation factor
45	1.0
35	1.5
25	2.0
15	2.5

An RPI greater than 3.0 suggests loss or accelerated destruction of RBCs. Note that the peak reticulocyte production occurs 3 to 5 days after an acute bleed.

  5. Blood chemistries may be helpful in evaluating certain types of anemias. Lactate dehydrogenase (LDH) and bilirubin, for example, are useful when considering hemolysis.

C. Treatment.

With acute blood loss, volume replacement is the primary concern. With massive losses (>2.5–3.0 L), red cell replacement (that is, blood transfusion) becomes important. It is generally more economical and effective to use packed RBCs for blood transfusion or packed RBCs and crystalloid for volume replacement. Most patients can tolerate a Hg as low as 8.0 (Hct of 24) and in many chronic conditions even lower than this. Certain patients, especially those with cardiovascular disease, do not tolerate as low an Hg; these individuals generally need a Hg of at least 10. Therefore any individual with symptoms from anemia, such as angina, congestive heart failure, profound fatigue, syncope, or persistent tachycardia, should receive a transfusion. Necessary blood tests should be obtained before transfusion. This is particularly important for iron studies, for the reticulocyte count (a transfusion can rapidly suppress the bone marrow response to an anemia), and for immunologic studies in hemolytic states.

II. Anemia: specific syndromes.

  A. Microcytic anemias.

These anemias generally reflect disorders of iron availability or utilization, or disorders of hemoglobin production. Nuclear maturation precedes hemoglobin incorporation, and the cells are small (microcytic) with a low concentration of hemoglobin (hypochromic). Iron studies are used to help differentiate these conditions (Table 6–2).

    1. Iron deficiency. This is the most common cause of anemia worldwide.

      a. Etiology: dietary insufficiency, impaired absorption (celiac disease, achlorhydria), increased requirements (pregnancy), increased losses (bleeding, menorrhagia, hemoglobinuria). Two or more of these factors may coexist (pregnancy and dietary insufficiency for example).

      b. Diagnosis: iron deficiency progresses through stages. First, low iron stores with no anemia, then a normocytic anemia, and finally a microcytic anemia. Therefore, approximately 30% of all iron deficiency anemias will be normocytic. Iron deficiency is associated with an increased RDW, unlike the thalassemias, which are usually associated with a normal RDW. Iron, total iron binding capacity (TIBC), and ferritin (Fe) are most commonly used in diagnosis (Table 6–3). Note that an Fe/TIBC of less than

TABLE 6–2.
Microcytic Anemias

Type of Anemia	Serum Iron (65–125 g/dL)	TIBC (265–350 g/dL)	%SAT 25%–40%	Ferritin (16–395 mg/mL)	Bone Marrow Iron
Iron deficiency*	<65	Normal	<15	2–8	No stainable iron
Anemia of chronic disease	Normal	Normal	Normal	Normal	Iron in marrow histiocytes but not in sideroblasts
Sideroblastic anemia	Normal	Normal	Normal	Normal	Ringed sideroblast
β-Thalassemia	Normal	Normal	Normal	Normal	Normal

*Most common.

TABLE 6–3.
Differential Diagnosis of Microcytic Hypochromic*

	Iron-Deficiency Anemia†	β-Thalassemia Trait	Anemia of Chronic Disease†	Sideroblastic Anemia
Serum iron	↓	N	↓	↑
TIBC	↑	N	↓	N
Serum ferritin	↓	N	↑	↑

*Adapted from Schafer A, Bunn F, in Braunwald E, et al (eds): Harrison's Principles of Internal Medicine, ed 11. New York, McGraw-Hill Book Co.
† ↑ = increased; ↓ = decreased; N = normal; TIBC = serum iron binding capacity.

10% can be very suggestive of the diagnosis of iron deficiency. A bone marrow aspirate demonstrating absent stainable iron remains the gold standard for diagnosis.

c. Treatment: consists of replenishing iron stores. Oral supplements include ferrous sulfate (the cheapest), ferrous gluconate and fumarate (better tolerated), and sustained release preparations (expensive, but well tolerated). Oral supplements are generally continued for 6 months, or until the ferritin level is normal. Parenteral replacement is generally reserved for patients who cannot tolerate or do not absorb oral medications. Iron given intramuscularly (can cause skin discoloration) or intravenously (can cause anaphylaxis) in the form of iron dextran. Dosage is determined by the iron deficit:

Iron deficit (mg) = body weight (kg) × [16 −
Hg (g/dL) + 600 (women) or 1,000 (men)].

2. Thalassemias. These are a group of congenital disorders characterized by a decreased production of one of the peptides comprising the hemoglobin molecule, either the α chains (α-thalassemia) or the β chains (β-thalassemia).

a. Classification: α-thalassemia is characterized by an absence of production of any or all of its four gene products, and hence there are four types of α-thalassemia depending on the number of genes affected: silent carrier, α-thalassemia trait, HbH disease, and hydrops fetalis. There are, however, only two genes coding for the β chain, and hence two major types of β-thalassemia: heterozygous (or β-thalassemia ss minor), and homozygous (or β-thalassemia major, Cooley's anemia).

    b. Diagnosis:

        1. Severe forms of thalassemia are almost always diagnosed in childhood and characterized either by fetal death or by a severe transfusion-dependent anemia, growth retardation, and skeletal deformities.

        2. Less severe forms of thalassemia are usually asymptomatic and characterized by a mild anemia with a very low MCV (55–70). RDW is usually normal.

        3. Hemoglobin electrophesis can be used to diagnose β-thalassemia. α-thalassemia has a normal hemoglobin electrophoresis, and is usually a diagnosis of exclusion.

        4. Definitive diagnosis of either can be made by gene mapping or globin-chain synthesis studies, but these are expensive and time-consuming and not readily available.

3. Anemia of chronic disease. This is a group of anemias associated with chronic inflammatory disorders.

    a. Etiology: this disorder is associated with a defect in iron utilization; the RBCs are unable to incorporate iron present within the bone marrow. The red cells may also have a shortened life span. These anemias are associated with chronic inflammatory conditions, such as infections (endocarditis, osteomyelitis, abcesses, tuberculosis, etc.), neoplasms (lymphomas, breast cancer, lung cancer, etc.), and rheumatologic diseases. These anemias are distinguished from anemias associated with other chronic, noninflammatory conditions such as uremia, endocrine failure, or liver disease. Chronic disease per se is not enough to cause this anemia; it must be a disease associated with inflammation.

b. Diagnosis: this anemia is generally normochromic and normocytic, and usually associated with a Hg greater than 8 g/dL. Thirty percent may be microcytic; however, rarely with an MCV below 70. Iron studies are generally used for diagnosis (Table 6–2), but the bone marrow aspirate is considered the gold standard and demonstrates an increase in stainable iron.

c. Treatment: treatment of the underlying disease.

4. Sideroblastic anemias. This is a group of diseases characterized by defective heme porphyrin synthesis and incorporation. There are many causes, which include drugs, inherited disorders, and neoplasia. They generally manifest a microcytic, hypochromic anemia and at least 10% ringed sideroblasts (RBC precursors with iron deposition within the mitochondria lying in a ring around the center of the cells) within the bone marrow.

B. Macrocytic anemias.

These anemias generally reflect disorders of nuclear maturation, cytoplasmic maturation precedes nuclear maturation, and the cells are large. It is important to distinguish megaloblastic macrocytic anemias associated with nuclear morphologic changes from normoblastic macrocytic anemias in which the nuclear morphology is generally normal.

1. Megaloblastic anemia. These anemias are characterized by impaired DNA synthesis. Generally seen are hypersegmented polymorphonuclear cells (>5 lobed nuclei) on the peripheral smear and megaloblastic changes

in the bone marrow (bizarre nuclear morphology and delayed nuclear maturation). Also characteristic is ineffective erythropoiesis with intramedullary hemolysis of these abnormal RBC precursors. Other rapidly dividing cell lines are also affected, and pancytopenia and changes in the skin and GI tract are not uncommon.

  a. Etiology:

     i. Folate deficiency from decreased ingestion or absorption (alcohol, malabsorption, or poor nutrition), or associated with increased requirements (hemolytic disorders or malignancies).

     ii. B12 deficiency is most frequently associated with pernicious anemia, but may also be caused by malabsorption and nutritional deficiencies.

     iii. Pernicious anemia is an autoimmune disease associated with antibodies against the gastric parietal cell and against intrinsic factor. These patients do not produce intrinsic factor and are unable to absorb vitamin B12. Pernicious anemia is associated invariably with atrophic gastritis.

     iv. Malignancy and disordered growth. Megaloblastic changes may be seen with leukemias and myelodysplastic disorders.

     v. Many drugs are associated with megaloblastic changes, particulary those that affect the purine or pyrimidine metabolic pathways, and include such drugs as zidovudine (AZT), 5-fluorouracil (5-FU), 6-mercaptopurine (6-MP), 6-thioguanine (6-TG), and azathioprine.

  b. Diagnosis:

     i. Folate deficiency: glossitis, high serum

LDH, and low serum folate and RBC
folate levels. The serum folate may
rapidly normalize with adequate nutrition; the RBC folate is therefore a more
accurate reflection of previous folate
deficiency.

ii. B12 deficiency: glossitis, high LDH,
neurologic symptoms are variable (loss
of proprioception, vibratory loss, optic
atrophy, mental status changes); pernicious anemia may also be associated
with other autoimmune disorders such
as vitiligo, thyrotoxicosis, Hashimoto's
thyroditis, etc. Serum B12 is low. Pernicious anemia can be diagnosed with
the Schilling's test.

c. Treatment:
Repletion of B12 or folic acid results in a
rapid hematologic response. In B12 deficiency, a partial response to folic acid may
be seen, but neurologic symptoms may be
worsened or precipitated. Transfusion in
these anemias may precipitate severe
congestive heart failure, and should be used
sparingly and extremely cautiously. Beware
of hypokalemia with replacement of B12 or
folic acid.

2. Normoblastic macrocytic anemias. These are a
diverse group of anemias and may be seen with
alcohol (independent of associated folate deficiency), hypothyroidism, chronic liver disease,
malignancies, and hemolytic disorders (also independent of folate deficiency).

C. Normocytic normochromic anemias.
These too are a diverse group of anemias with many
causes:

1. Acute bleeding: maximal reticulocyte response
occurs 3 to 5 days later.

2. Anemia of chronic disease: discussed under mi-

crocytic anemias. Approximately 70% of these are normochromic.

3. Inadequate blood formation of various types: myelophthistic anemia (discussed below), hypoplastic anemias, and aplastic anemias.

4. Endocrine diseases: hypothyroidism, hyperthyroidism, hypopituitarism, and hypogonadism.

5. Chronic renal failure: associated with inadequate erythropoietin and decreased RBC survival.

6. Hemolysis: to be discussed.

D. Hemolytic anemias.

RBC lysis occurs either intravascularly or, more commonly, extravascularly (within the bone marrow or the reticuloendothelial system). These anemias are classified in general as defects of the RBC membrane (either primary or secondary), as cytoplasmic disorders (enzymatic defects or hemoglobinopathies), or as toxin- or immune-mediated cell lysis.

1. Diagnosis (general).

Diagnosis of hemolysis in general rests on the demonstration of three areas of abnormalities:

a. Increased marrow response: polychromasia, increased reticulocyte count, and RPI.

b. Destruction of red cells with cellular release:

i. Morphologic abnormalities: spherocytes, sickled cells, fragmented cells (schistocytes and helmet-cells).

ii. Released cellular contents: increased serum bilirubin, increased serum LDH (primarily fractions 1 and 2), free serum hemoglobin, decreased serum haptoglobin, and increased urinary free hemoglobin and hemosiderin.

c. Shortened RBC survival times measured by chromium-labeled RBC survival studies. These studies are occasionally needed to

    confirm hemolysis and may be useful for
    quantitating the degree of hemolysis.

2. Treatment.

  a. Folic acid should be given in all hemolytic
     disorders.

  b. In general, iron is not indicated and may
     actually contribute to iron overload. How-
     ever, urinary iron loss may occur with brisk
     intravascular hemolysis, and iron supple-
     mentation may occasionally be needed.

  c. Transfusions should be avoided, especialy
     in cases of autoimmune hemolysis.

3. Etiology.

  a. Membrane defects are in general uncom-
     mon, and include hereditary spherocytosis,
     hereditary elliptocytosis, stomatocytosis,
     acanthocytosis, and paroxysmal nocturnal
     hemoglobinuria.

  b. Enzymopathies: either of the glycolytic or
     the hexose monophosphate shunt pathways:

    1. Pyruvate kinase deficiency is the most
       common (95%) of the uncommon gly-
       colytic pathway defects. Hexokinase
       deficiency is the next most common.

    2. Glucose-6-phosphate dehydrogenase
       (G6PD) deficiency is the only common
       enzymopathy and is associated with
       hemolysis during oxidant stress in the
       face of inadequate glutathione stores. It
       is seen in up to 10% of the black popu-
       lation (usually mild) and in the Medi-
       terranean and oriental populations (less
       common but more severe). Hemolysis
       is seen with infections, or with various
       drugs or toxins (such as antimalarials,
       sulfonamides, etc.). The diagnosis is
       suspected by hemolysis in the right
       clinical setting, and confirmed with
       measurement of G6PD levels obtained
       after periods of hemolysis.

   c. Hemoglobinopathies including hemoglobin C disease, sickle cell disease, sickle thalassemia disease, and other less common disorders. Sickle cell anemia or hemoglobin S disease is by far the most common.

     1. Etiology: sickle cell syndromes occur with inherited gene defects in the hemoglobin molecule that are associated with sickling of the affected RBCs, causing hemolysis and vaso-occlusion.

     2. Complications:

        i. Hemolysis is usually constant, but worse with infections and stress.

        ii. Vaso-occlusive crises are the typical painful crises of sickle cell anemia, are distinct from hemolysis, and arise from tissue sludging of the sickled cells.

        iii. Aplastic crisis is caused by nutritional deficiencies or viral infections (parvovirus most classically). Heralded by a decreasing reticulocyte response and worsening anemia.

        iv. Specific organ dysfunction or damage from vaso-occlusion includes: pulmonary infarction, splenic sequestration crisis, osteonecrosis and osteomyelitis, legs ulcers, priapism, gallstones, and renal dysfunction (papillary necrosis, decreased tubular function).

     3. Diagnosis: sickle cell disorders usually present in childhood, and in general are suspected clinically. Hemoglobin electrophoresis demonstrates an abnormal hemoglobin molecule. Gene mapping studies of fetal blood can be used for prenatal diagnosis.

4. Treatment:
    i. General: pneumococcal vaccine (frequent sequestration crises and infarction cause functional asplenia), daily folic acid, oral pain medication, and hydration. Exchange transfusions are indicated for frequent and severe pain crises, for life-threatening complications, and preoperatively (to get HgS below 50%).
    ii. Pain crises: hydration, correction of electrolyte abnormalities, treatment of hypoxemia, parenteral analgesia, and adequate nutrition are important. Reticulocyte counts should be followed up for aplastic crisis. Infection should be ruled out (WBC count is often elevated by the pain crisis alone). Transfusions are not effective for treating pain crises, but are useful for prevention.
  d. Immune-mediated hemolytic anemias are a group of disorders in which red cell destruction results from the binding and interaction of immunoglobulins and complement on the red cell surface. Hemolysis may be intra- or extravascular.
    1. Etiology: Antibodies may be cold-reacting (generally IgM) or they may be warm-reacting (IgG). Complement is generally seen with IgM-related hemolysis and is more frequently associated with intravascular hemolysis. Antibodies may occur secondary to other disorders (SLE, lymphomas and leukemias, infections, or various drugs) or they may occur as the primary disorder.
    2. Diagnosis: typical features of hemolysis

discussed above are seen. Demonstration of antibodies and complement on the RBC surface is generally confirmatory (direct antiglobin test, *direct Coombs*). Antibodies may also be found in the serum itself (indirect antiglobin test, *indirect Coombs*).

3. Treatment: mild hemolysis may require no therapy. More severe cases generally require glucocorticoids initially in high doses. In some cases immunosuppression (azathioprine or cyclophosphamide) may be needed.

e. Drugs and chemicals: many drugs can cause hemolysis by several different mechanisms, including immune-mediated Coombs' positive reactions (penicillins, cephalosporins, methyldopa, quinidine) and direct toxic effects (copper, arsenic, and various simple organic compounds).

f. Parasites: intracellular parasites causing hemolysis include malaria, babesiosis, and bartonellosis.

g. Trauma: ''march hemoglobinuria,'' cardiac abnormalities (especially valvular heart disease), and trauma within the microcirculation (microangiopathic hemolytic anemia) may all cause mechanical disruption of the red cells with lysis. The peripheral smear will show signs of red cell fragmentation (schistocytes and helmet cells). Microangiopathic hemolytic anemia may be seen with DIC, with TTP, and with various diffuse vascular disorders such as malignancies, hemangiomas, vasculitis, and malignant hypertension.

E. Aplastic anemia.

This is a disorder characterized by primary failure of blood precursors associated with pancytopenia. Anemia is only one manifestation.

1. Etiology: 50% of cases are idiopathic. The rest are of various other causes: viral infections (especially non-A non-B hepatitis, Epstein Barr virus, and Parvovirus); and drug related, either dose dependent and predictable (cytosine arabinoside, busulfan, etc.) or idiosyncratic (chloramphenicol, phenylbutazone, gold, quinacrine, organic arsenicals, and benzene).

2. Diagnosis: pancytopenia must be differentiated with a bone marrow aspirate or biopsy from leukemias and myelodysplastic syndromes and from myelophthistic processes. Severe aplastic anemia is associated with:

   a. Anemia with a RPI <1.

   b. Neutropenia (neutrophils $<500/mm^3$).

   c. Thrombocytopenia (platelet count $<20,000/mm^3$).

   d. Bone marrow with $<25\%$ cellularity.

3. Treatment:

   a. Bone marrow transplantation is the treatment of choice for those with available donors. Durable complete responses can be seen in 70% to 80% of transplantations. Lower responses are seen in previously transfused patients; patients who will or may receive a transplant should not receive a transfusion unless necessary.

   b. Anti-lymphocyte globulin (ALG) or anti-thymocyte globulin (ATG) are useful for those patients who are unsuitable for transplantation. Response rates of 60% can be attained.

   c. General guidelines include transfusion therapy when needed, antibiotic therapy for fever, suppression of menstruation in females, and avoidance of aspirin and anti-platelet agents.

F. Myelofibrosis and myelophthistic anemias.
   These are anemias that follow the replacement or fi-

brosis of the bone marrow and are characterized by extramedullary hematopoeisis.

1. Etiology:
   a. Malignancies: leukemia, lymphoma, plasma cell neoplasms, or metastatic solid tumors (lung, breast, prostate, stomach).
   b. Replacement by tuberculosis or fungal infections, or by lipid storage diseases (Gaucher's disease, etc.).
   c. Myelofibrosis: primary (myelofibrosis with myeloid metaplasia) or secondary (any of the myeloproliferative diseases may cause myelofibrosis, as well as several cytotoxic and chemotherapeutic agents).

2. Diagnosis:
   a. Fibrosis or infiltration of the bone marrow as demonstrated with a bone marrow aspirate (frequently inaspirable) or biopsy. Reticulin stains should routinely be ordered with special stains (AFB, silver stain for fungus, etc.) as indicated clinically.
   b. Extramedullary hematopoiesis with early forms in the periphery seen usually only in the bone marrow (leukoerythroblastosis), such as nucleated RBCs, myelocytes, myeloblasts, and giant platelets.

3. Treatment: treatment of the underlying disorder. Myelofibrosis with myeloid metaplasia is poorly responsive to chemotherapy. Treatment is supportive and androgens have occasionally been effective.

BIBLIOGRAPHY

Hematologic Disease

Williams WJ: *Textbook of Hematology*, ed 3. New York, McGraw Hill Book Co, 1983.
Wyngaarden JB, Smith LH: *Cecil Textbook of Medicine*, ed 17. Philadelphia, WB Saunders Co, 1985.

Oncology

Larry Cripe, M.D.
Mary Jacobs, M.D.

7

Anticipation, recognition, and treatment of the complications of advanced carcinoma and its therapy are important contributions to the care of the patient with cancer.

I. Complications of Advanced Carcinoma.
   A. Cardiovascular.
      1. Pericardial effusion.
         a. Most commonly occurs with lung and breast cancer, sarcomas, melanoma, and lymphoma.
         b. Presents with dyspnea, orthopnea, cough, pericarditis, edema; most are asymptomatic.
         c. Signs: edema, jugular venous distention, hepatomegaly, cyanosis, pulsus paradoxus, and Kussmauls' sign (neck vein distension that increases with inspiration).
         d. Therapy: Pericardiocentesis if hypotensive; chemotherapy or radiation may be palliative.
      2. Superior vena cava obstruction.
         a. Ninety percent of cases have either associated lung carcinoma or lymphoma.
         b. Usually an insidious presentation with dyspnea, facial edema, pain, and lethargy.
         c. Signs: thoracic and neck vein distension associated with facial edema. Chest x-ray demonstrates a mass in 90% of cases.
         d. Local radiation therapy or chemotherapy are recommended treatments.
      3. Venous obstruction is not always due to intra-

vascular thrombosis, and extrinsic compression should be ruled out.

B. Pulmonary.

   1. Pleural effusions.

      a. Malignant effusions are most commonly due to lung and breast carcinoma or lymphoma; 5% are due to gastrointestinal (GI) or genitourinary cancers.

      b. Patients present with cough, chest pain, or dyspnea; as many as 25% are asymptomatic.

      c. Thoracentesis will yield positive cytologic findings in 40% to 50%; multiple samples increase the yield to 90%.

      d. Treatment with thoracentesis and systemic chemotherapy may prevent recurrence. If the effusion does recur, chest tube drainage with pleurodesis (Bleomycin or tetracycline sclerotherapy) is recommended.

C. Hepatic metastatic disease.

   1. Very common site of metastases, especially for GI or pancreatic tumors.

   2. May be asymptomatic, or jaundice, pruritus, abdominal discomfort, and biliary obstruction may be the initial presentation.

   3. Hepatic involvement is a poor prognostic factor.

D. Metabolic complications of carcinoma.

   1. SIADH (see Renal).

   2. Ectopic ACTH (see Endocrine).

   3. Hypercalcemia.

      a. Most commonly seen with breast, lung, multiple myeloma, and head and neck carcinoma. Rare with leukemia-lymphoma (unless HTLV-I associated).

      b. Symptoms: anorexia, nausea, constipation, polyuria, polydipsia, and confusion.

      c. Treatment.

         i. Hydration and furosemide: aim for a urinary output of 250 mL/hr.

         ii. Mithramycin: Recommended for refractory cases (25 μg/kg intravenously

every 4 days; effect in 24 to 48 hours).
Avoid with hepatic disease. Lower dose
(10 μg/kg) in renal failure.

iii. Calcitonin: 3 to 6 μ/kg intravenous infusion over 24 hours or 150 μ subcutaneously every 12 hours. Effect seen in 2 to 4 hours.

iv. Corticosteroids are especially useful in multiple myeloma.

v. Diphosphonates: Enhances transfer of calcium into bone.

E. Adrenal insufficiency.

Many of the symptoms of advanced malignancy may simulate adrenal insufficiency: fever, lethargy, anorexia, low blood pressure, or eosinophilia. Consider this diagnosis.

F. Tumor lysis syndrome.

1. Is associated with hyperkalemia, hyperuricemia, hyperphosphatemia, and hypocalcemia after therapy of lymphoma, leukemia (especially Burkitts lymphoma). Uncommon with solid tumors.

2. Preventive measures include prehydration, urinary alkalinization, and allopurinal 24 hours prior to administration of chemotherapy.

3. Patients present with headaches, seizures, confusion, focal deficits, and obtundation.

4. Therapy: fluid and electrolyte management.

G. Meningeal involvement.

1. May present with involvement of multiple levels of the neuroaxis.

2. Cerebrospinal fluid evaluation of glucose, protein, cytologic studies usually reveal at least one abnormality.

3. Therapy includes dexamethosone and intrathecal chemotherapy: methotrexate, cytarabine, or thiotepa. This therapy should only be initiated under recommendations of an oncologist.

H. Marrow metastases.

Classic manifestation is leukoerythroblastosis, more commonly anemia and/or granulocytopenia and/or thrombocytopenia.

I. Skeletal metastases.
1. Eighty percent are from breast, lung, and prostate; 20% are from renal, thyroid, bladder, cervix, and multiple myeloma.
2. These metastases are frequently associated with bone pain (especially nocturnal), fractures, and hypercalcemia.
3. Local percussion tenderness.
4. Radiographic features include:
   a. Seventy percent occur in the axial skeleton.
   b. Osteolytic: breast, renal, thyroid, multiple myeloma; osteoblastic: breast or prostate.
5. Radiation therapy is effective especially for pain relief. Surgical stabilization may be required.

II. Organ system toxicity of systemic chemotherapeutic agents (Table 7–1).
A. Nausea.
1. Agents commonly associated with severe nausea and emesis.
   a. Nitrogen mustard in 3 to 6 hours; subsides by 36 hours.
   b. Dacarbazine (DTIC).
   c. Nitrosureas (BCNU, CCNU).
   d. Cisplatin: occurs in 1 to 6 hours, subsides in 24 hours, may persist 72 to 96 hours. Anorexia may exist for days to weeks.
2. Moderate or dose-dependent nausea.
   a. Cyclophosphamide.
   b. Doxorubicin (immediate at 45 mg/m^2).
   c. 5-FU especially with bolus injections.
   d. Methotrexate (rare with lower doses).
3. Therapy: a list of all common antiemetics is in the formulary.
   a. Choice of drug regimen varies with institution, chemotherapeutic agent, and the specific patient.

TABLE 7–1.
Toxicity of Chemotherapeutic Agents

Agent	Nausea Emesis	Myelosuppression	Mucositis	Renal	Other
Vincristine	–	±	±	–	Peripheral neuropathy
Vinblastine	–	++	+	–	Myalgias, constipation, fever,
Bleomycin	–	–	+++	–	Pulmonary fibrosis (>400U).
Adriamycin	++	+++	+	–	Cardiomyopathy (>550 mg/ m²).
Mitomycin	+	+	+	±	Long nadir/HUS
Actinomycin	±	+	–	–	Flu, acute cellular dysfunction
Ara/C	±	+	++	–	Corneal dryness, dizziness, cerebellar dysfunction
5-FU	+	+	++	–	Pulmonary, fever, cholestasis
Methotrexate	–	+	+++	+	
6 Mercaptopurine	+	+	+	–	
Nitrogen Mustard	+++ ++	+++ +	– +	– –	Tinnitus, hematuria, SIADH
Cyclophosphamide					
Chlorambucil	–	+	–	–	
Melphalan	+	+	–	–	Pulmonary fibrosis, long nadir
Nitrosureas	+	+	–	–	Pulmonary fibrosis
Hydroxyurea	–	++	±	–	Delayed hematologic toxicity:
Cisplatin	++++	+	±	+	Skin
VP16	–	+	–	–	Acute renal failure, ototoxicity
DTIC	+++	+	–	–	Fever, hypotension
					Flu syndrome

1. First line: Phenothiazines (Compazine) 10 mg orally or intravenously every 4 to 6 hours as needed. May need diphenhydramine chloride (Benadryl) 25 mg intravenously or 50 mg orally if a dystonic reaction to Compazine occurs.
2. Second line: dexamethasone (Decadron) 10–20 mg intravenously as a one-time dose prior to chemotherapy.
3. Third line: lorazepam (Ativan) 1–2 mg orally or intravenously every 6 hours as needed.
4. If platinum-containing regimen or refractory nausea: metoclopramide (Reglan) 2 mg/kg intravenously one-half hour prior to dose of chemotherapy and then every 2 hours intravenously for three to five doses.

B. Mucosal toxicity (Table 7–2).

The gastrointestinal epithelium is a rapidly proliferating tissue susceptible to chemotherapy. Stomatitis, glossitis, cheilitis, oral ulceration, esophagitis, and diarrhea may result. Always consider secondary infection by bacteria or opportunistic agents such as candida or herpes simplex virus.

1. Methotrexate.

Incidence and severity are dependent on dose, schedule, and proper use of leucovorin.

2. 5-FU.

Toxicity of weekly injection is less than daily continuous infusion. The patient may have bloody diarrhea.

3. Adriamycin, bleomycin, and vinblastine: associated mucositis may be severe and ulcerative. Adriamycin toxicity is worse if prior radiation therapy or liver disease (contraindicated) is present.

4. Ara-C has been associated with severe enteritis characterized by profuse diarrhea, hemorrhage, and perforation.

TABLE 7–2.
Treatment of Mucosal Side Effects of Chemotherapeutic Agents

Problem	Medication	Use
Oral candidiasis	Nystatin oral suspension	Rinse and swallow 300,000 U three to four times daily
	Clotrimazole troche 10 mg	Dissolve one tablet five times daily
Mucositis (generalized)	Xylocaine viscous 2% solution	15 mL every 2 to 3 hours, expectorate
	Dyclonine hydrochloride 0.5% or 1% solution	15 mL every 2 to 3 hours, expectorate
	Benadryl and Kaopectate mix solution of 50% each	15 mL for 2 to 3 hours, expectorate
Mucositis (localized)	Benzocaine in orabase ointment Kenalog in orabase ointment	Apply to affected dried area every 2 to 3 hours
Local Bleeding		
Gingival	Topical thrombin solution	Apply to affected area with gauze sponge and hold in place with pressure for 30 min. Do not remove formed clots.
Mucosal surface bleeding	Microfibrillar collagen	Apply to dried site with dry gauze sponge for 1 to 5 min; do not use in closure of mucosal incisions
Xerostomia		
Saliva substitutes	Salivary synthetic	Spray as needed
Saline	Saliva-spray	Rinse as needed

C. Hepatoxicity:
1. BCNU: mild increased elevation in SGOT, alkaline phosphatase, and bilirubin in 20% of patients at 1 to 18 weeks; usually transient.
2. 6-Mercaptopurine is associated with an elevation in liver enzymes resembling cholestasis.
3. Methotrexate.
   a. Cirrhosis may be associated with long-term use of a low dose.
   b. Acute hepatic necrosis is rare with high-dose, intermittent therapy.
4. Ara-C: transient mild cholestasis or SGOT/SGPT elevation.

D. Pulmonary toxicity.
Usually manifests as chronic pneumonitis, less commonly hypersensitivity lung disease or noncardiogenic pulmonary edema.
1. Bleomycin pulmonary toxicity occurs in approximately 4% of all treated patients and is lethal in 1%.
   a. Incidence is dose dependent.
   b. Risk factors: radiation therapy, uremia, and increased age may result in adverse effects at lower doses.
2. BCNU toxicity occurs in approximately 20% to 30% of patients.
   a. Symptoms may develop within 1 month.
   b. Possible synergistic toxicity with Cyclophosphamide.
3. Busulfan has approximately a 4% clinical toxicity.
   a. Usually at a dose of 500 mg or greater unless radiation therapy is used.
   b. Symptoms develop (evolve slowly) over 9 to 120 months.
4. Cyclophosphamide has approximately a 1% clinical toxicity.
   a. Usually present within 2 weeks.
   b. May be with only 200 mg/kg.

     5. Cytosine arabinoside (controversial) may cause noncardiogenic pulmonary edema.

     6. Chlorambucil, mitomycin, melphalan, methotrexate may produce chronic pneumonitis. Methotrexate has been associated with acute hypersensitivity reactions even with intrathecal therapy.

E. Skin toxicity.

     1. Methotrexate, Ara-C hydroxyurea: Erythematous, which is truncal, short-lived, and usually disappears.

     2. Bleomycin: raised, painful hyperkeratotic lesions on the distal extremities and pressure points.

     3. Busulfan: progressive generalized hyperpigmentation with long-term use.

     4. DTIC: phototoxicity.

     5. Adriamycin: local hyperpigmentation of nails and mucosa.

     6. Actinomycin D: recall folliculitis (erythema in previously irradiated areas).

F. Cardiovascular toxicity.

     1. Doxorubicin (Adriamycin).

        a. Reversible nonspecific ST wave changes, loss of voltage, supraventricular tachycardias in up to 40% of patients.

        b. Cardiomyopathy may occur in 10% of all patients and is associated with a 50% mortality rate.

        c. Low risk patients: less than 70 years old, no history of mediastinal irradiation, and no history of hypertension or underlying heart disease.

        d. Dose-dependent risk: 5% at 500 mg/m^2.

        e. Risk may be less for lower doses administered weekly.

        f. Observe for 30% increase in the QRS voltage, possible early signs of heart failure, and follow the ejection fraction with a MUGA scan.

2. Daunorubicin (daunomycin): side effects are similar to those of doxorubicin. Limit dose to 600–1000 mg/m^2.

3. Cyclophosphamide (Cytoxan): adverse effects are restricted to patients receiving massive doses; i.e., usually bone marrow transplant patients.

4. 5-FU: several cases of myocardial ischemia 3 to 18 hours after injection have been described.

5. Cisplatin: ischemic arterial disease (Raynauds, cerebral vascular accidents, myocardial infarction).

G. Renal toxicity.

1. Methotrexate: primary route of elimination is renal excretion.
   a. Renal damage is dose-dependent.
      i. Ameliorated by brisk diuresis and urinary alkalinization.
      ii. Methotrexate not cleared effectively with peritoneal or hemodialysis.
      iii. Renal failure usually resolves within 2 to 3 weeks.

2. Cisplatin.
   a. Proximal tubular damage is common, and may be reduced by infusion rather than bolus therapy, and maintenance of adequate urine flow rates.
   b. Permanent severe dysfunction is rare.
   c. Associated with hyperuricemia, hypomagnesemia, and hypocalcemia.

3. Cyclophosphamide.
   a. Hematuria secondary to bladder mucosal toxicity: maintain urine flow and frequent voiding.
   b. Hyponatremia at doses of 50 mg/kg secondary to impaired water excretion (SIADH).

4. Mitomycin C.
   Associated with the hemolytic uremic syndrome.

5. Nitrosureas (CCNU + BCNU).
   a. Progressive glomerosclerosis at high total doses.
   b. Twenty-six percent incidence if dose greater than 1400 mg/m^2.

H. Neurotoxicity.
   1. Methotrexate (intrathecal Ara-C has similar toxicity).
      a. Two to four hours after intrathecal administration: stiff neck, headache, lethargy, fever, cerebrospinal fluid pleocytosis; lasting 12 to 72 hours.
      b. Transient paraplegia.
      c. Encephalopathy.
   2. Cisplatin.
      a. Ototoxicity: tinnitus, high frequency loss related to cumulative dose.
      b. Bilateral symmetric sensory neuropathy; rarely motor dysfunction (after three to four doses or total dose of 210–825 mg/m^2).
      c. Papilledema and retrobulbar neuritis.
   3. Vincristine.
      a. Peripheral neuropathy.
         Symmetric motor dysfunction and sensory symptoms are prominent; loss of deep tendon reflexes.
      b. Autonomic neuropathy.
         Constipation, colicky abdominal pain, orthostatic hypotension, bladder atony (rare).
   4. 5-FU.
      Acute cerebellar syndrome.

I. Hematologic (Table 7–3).

J. Extravasation injuries.
   1. Extravasation.
      Defined as the leakage of a vesicant or irritant drug into subcutaneous tissue that is capable of causing pain, necrosis and/or sloughing of tis-

TABLE 7-3.
Hematologic Toxicity

Agent	WBC	Platelets	Peak effect (Days)	Recovery (Days)
For which myelosuppression is dose limiting				
Vinblastine	+ +	+	5–9	14–21
Mechlorethamine	+ +	+	7–15	28
Melphalan	+	+	10–12	42–50
Busulfan	+	+	11–30	24–54
Chlorambucil	+	+	14–28	28–42
Nitrosoureas	+ +	+	28–63	35–91
ARA-C	+	+	12–14	22–24
VP16	+	+	16	20
For which myelosuppression is accompanied by other serious side effects				
Cyclophosphamide	+	±	8–14	18–25
Methotrexate	+	+	7–14	14–21
Hydroxurea	+	+	18–30	21–35
Mitomycin	+	+ + +	28–42	42–56
Mithramycin	±	+ +	14	21–28
Actinomycin	+ +	+ +	14–21	22–25
Adriamycin	+ +	±	10–14	21–24
DTIC	+	+	21–28	28–35
For which myelosuppression is not dose limiting				
Vincristine	+	+	4–5	7
Bleomycin	+	+	–	–
Cisplatin	+	+	14	21

sue. Vesicant drugs are capable of forming a blister and causing tissue destruction. Causative agents include: dactinomycin, mitomycin C, DTIC, nitrogen mustard, daunomycin, vinblastine, adriamycin, vincristine, mithramycin (high dose), and amsacrine (m-amsa). Irritant drugs are capable of producing venous pain at the site or along the vein with or without associated inflammation.

2. Treatment:
   a. Stop chemotherapeutic agent and leave needle in place.
   b. Aspirate residual drug and blood in intravenous tubing, needle, and suspected site.
   c. If drug has an intravenous antidote, instill and remove needle. If unable to aspirate residual drug, then just remove needle and continue with step d.
   d. If drug has a subcutaneous antidote, remove needle and inject antidote clockwise into infiltrated area with a 25-G needle. Change needle with each new injection.
   e. Do not apply pressure to suspected site.
   f. Photograph site and cover with occlusive sterile dressing.
   g. Apply warm compresses as required.
   h. Keep arm elevated and consider plastic surgery if early.

BIBLIOGRAPHY

Dorr RT: *Cancer Chemotherapy Handbook.* London, Henry Kimpton Publishers Ltd, 1980.

Yarbro JW, Bernstein R: *Oncologic Emergencies.* Philadelphia, Grune & Stratton, 1980.

Oncology Nursing Society: *Cancer Chemotherapy. Guidelines and Recommendations for Nursing Education and Practice.* Pittsburgh, Oncology Nursing Society, 1984.

Perry MC, ed: Toxicity of chemotherapy. Sem Oncol 1983; 9:1–154.

Rheumatology

Rosemarie Jeffrey, M.D.

I. Mechanisms of inflammation and tissue destruction. Inflammatory processes play a major role in the pathogenesis of rheumatic diseases. Mediators of inflammation include arachidonic acid metabolites, histamine, serotonin, complement cleavage products, kinins, interleukins, and lysosomal enzymes (Table 8–1).

II. Rheumatologic disorders.

    A. Crystal-induced arthropathies.

        1. Gout.

            a. Etiology: gouty attacks require the deposition of monosodium urate crystals in the joint. The deposition occurs in the setting of an elevated serum uric acid level.

            b. Presentation: gout usually presents as an acute, very painful monoarthritis (acute gouty arthritis). Commonly afflicted joints include the first metatarsophalangeal joints, tarsal joints, ankles, heels, and knees. The disease can progress over a period of years to polyarticular involvement with the formation of subcutaneous deposits of monosodium urate crystals called tophi (tophaceous gout).

            c. Diagnosis: diagnosis depends on the demonstration of strongly negative birefringent needle-shaped crystals (monosodium urate monohydrate) in the synovial fluid of a clinically active joint, or from a tophaceous deposit.

            d. Treatment: there are two parts to treatment.

TABLE 8–1.
Types of Immunologically Mediated Inflammation*

Type of Inflammation	Recognition Component	Soluble Mediator	Inflammatory Response	Disease Example
I Reagenic, allergic	IgE	Basophil and mast cell products	Immediate flare and wheal smooth muscle constriction	Atopy, anaphylaxis
II Cytotoxic antibody	IgG, IgM	Complement	Lysis or phagocytosis of circulating antigens, acute inflammation in tissues	Autoimmune hemolytic anemia, thrombocytopenia associated with systemic lupus erythematosus
III Immune complex	IgG, IgM	Complement	Accumulation of polymorphonuclear leukocytes and macrophages	Rheumatoid arthritis, lupus erythematosus
IV Delayed hypersensitivity	T lymphocytes	Cytokines	Mononuclear cell infiltrate	Tuberculosis, sarcoidosis, polymyositis, granulomatosis, vasculitis

*Adapted from Synderman R: Mechanisms of inflammation and tissue destruction in the rheumatic diseases, in Wyngaarden JB, Smith LH (eds): *Cecil Textbook of Medicine.* Philadelphia, WB Saunders Co, 1985; p 1903. Used by permission.

First is the reduction of inflammation to help the patient through the acute flare. This can be done with nonsteroidal anti-inflammatory drugs (NSAIDs), oral colchicine, or steroids (e.g., intramuscular adrenocorticotrophic hormone). Second is to reduce the serum uric acid level with allopurinol or, in appropriate patients, with a uricosuric agent.

2. Pseudogout or calcium pyrophosphate deposition disease (CPPD).
   a. Etiology: deposition of calcium pyrophosphate crystals within the joint.
   b. Presentation: pseudogout can present much like gout, but most commonly affects the knees. Almost any other synovial joint can be involved. Pseudogout can also present as a polyarthritis, and can mimic rheumatoid arthritis. It can be associated with diseases such as osteoarthritis, hyperparathyroidism, hemochromatosis, and hypothyroidism.
   c. Diagnosis: diagnosis depends on the demonstration of weakly positive birefringent rhomboidal crystals in the synovial fluid of a clinically involved joint. Corroborative evidence of CPPD is the finding of chondrocalcinosis on radiographs of affected joints.
   d. Treatment: NSAIDs have proven quite effective. Joint aspiration followed by intraarticular steroid injections can provide good pain relief.

B. Osteoarthritis.
   1. Etiology: probably multifactorial with genetics and mechanical stresses playing roles.
   2. Presentation: generally, there is little inflammation evident compared to that of crystal arthropathies or rheumatoid arthritis. Local pain with joint usage is usually the initial complaint. Three common initial presentations are:

      a. Pain and stiffness of large joints such as the hips or knees in an elderly or middle-aged person. Joint involvement is frequently asymmetric.

      b. Firm nodular swellings of the distal interphalangeal joints (DIPs) called Heberden's nodes, and of the proximal interphalangeal joints (PIPs) called Bouchard's nodes.

      c. Osteoarthritis of the spine can present as neck or lower back pain and radiculopathies.

  3. Diagnosis: made on the basis of clinical presentation, the finding of noninflammatory synovial fluid from an affected joint, and characteristic radiographic signs.

  4. Treatment: weight loss can be helpful in obese patients when weight-bearing joints are affected. Physical therapy including local heat treatments and range of motion exercises is beneficial. Aspirin and NSAIDs are mainstays of initial therapy. Intraarticular steriod injections, used sparingly, can help many patients.

     Total prosthetic joint replacements can relieve pain and restore mobility to patients with severe hip or knee disease.

C. Rheumatoid arthritis (RA).

  1. Etiology: presumably immunogenic. Rheumatoid factor, or IgM directed against the Fc portion of human or animal IgG can be found in the serum of 70% of patients.

  2. Presentation: symmetric, inflammatory polyarthritis characteristically involving the metacarpophalangeal (MCP) joints, the PIP joints, the metatarsophalangeal (MTP) joints, and the wrists, ankles, knees, hips, and shoulders. Affected joints will be warm and swollen. Spongy synovial swelling and tenderness is evident on palpation. Morning stiffness in untreated disease generally lasts more than 30 minutes and

can last for hours. Systemic signs such as fatigue and weight loss are frequently present. Extraarticular manifestations include subcutaneous nodules, pleural effusions, pulmonary infiltrates, vasculitis, and Sjögrens Syndrome. As the disease progresses, characteristic deformities of the joints may develop. These include ulnar deviation of the fingers, including boutonniere and swan-neck deformities.

3. Diagnosis: American Rheumatism Association diagnostic criterian for RA include continuous symmetric involvement of tender, swollen joints for at least 6 weeks. Other criteria include subcutaneous nodules, characteristic radiographic and synovial fluid findings, and rheumatoid factor. Many patients with RA will not fulfill the diagnostic criteria for classic or definite RA at the time of initial presentation.

4. Treatment: a full discussion of treatment is beyond the scope of this text. Therapy is initiated with patient education about the disease and about joint protection techniques, rest, occupational and physical therapy. NSAIDs, or high-dose aspirin therapy are first line treatments. If synovitis cannot be alleviated with these measures or if the patient developes radiographic bone erosions, more aggressive therapy is indicated. More aggressive agents for RA include steroids, intramuscular or oral gold, D-penicillamine, azathioprine, and methotrexate.

D. Systemic lupus erythematosis (SLE).

1. Etiology is presumably immunologic. Antinuclear antibodies (ANAs) and immune complexes can be found serologically, and vasculitis and immune complex deposits can be found histopathologically.

2. Presentation and epidemiology.

   a. Women are affected eight times more often than men. In the United States, prevalence in black women is almost three times that in white women. SLE most often afflicts adolescents and young adults, but children and the elderly can also be afflicted.

b. SLE can have a variety of presentations depending on which organ systems are initially involved. A typical presentation might be a young woman with fatigue, low grade fevers, arthralgias, and a rash.

3. Diagnosis:

a. A firm diagnosis of SLE can be made when four of 11 American Rheumatism Association criteria are met in the absence of other likely causes of these abnormalities. The 11 criteria are: malar rash; discoid rash; photosensitivity-skin rash as a result of an unusual reaction to sunlight; oral or nasopharyngeal ulceration; nonerosive arthritis; serositis-pleuritis or pericarditis; renal insufficiency and/or abnormal urinary sediment; neurologic disorder-seizures or psychosis; hematologic disorder-hemolytic anemia with reticulocytosis, leukopenia, or lymphopenia, or thrombocytopenia; immunologic disorder (positive LE prep, anti-native DNA, Anti-SM, or false-positive results on a serologic test for syphilis; and antinuclear anti-body.

b. Other clinical features include Raynaud's phenomenon, alopecia, retinal cytoid bodies, and Sjögren's syndrome.

4. Treatment: the clinical manifestations are quite variable. Mild arthralgias can be treated with aspirin, NSAIDs, or hydroxychloroquine. Severe serositis, small vessel vasculitis, arthritis, and some renal lesions require adrenal corticosteroids. Life-threatening manifestations require high-dose pulse steroids and sometimes cytotoxic agents such as cyclophosphamide or aza-

thioprine. These manifestations include focal proliferative glomerulonephritis and neurologic disease such as seizures, alteration in consciousness, aseptic meningitis, and transverse myelitis.

E. Spondyloarthropathies (Table 8–2).

   1. Etiology: there is a genetic predisposition with markedly increased frequency of HLA-B27 in this group of patients.

   2. Presentation: is frequently sacroiliac and back pain which is worse in the morning and improves with movement. Morning stiffness is prominent. More peripheral joints can also be affected; e.g., hips, shoulders, or knees. Men tend to be more severely affected than women. There are several spondyloarthropathies.

     a. Ankylosing spondylitis: over 90% of these patients have HLA B27. The disease can progress to bony ankylosis of the spine, resulting in a rigid, fused vertebral column.

     b. Reiter's syndrome: the classic triad of Reiter's syndrome, urethritis, conjunctivitis, and arthritis, can follow venereal urethritis in the appropriate host. Over 90% of these patients have HLA B27. The arthritis characteristically affects weight-bearing joints including the sacroiliac joints and vertebral column. Other findings include periostitis, keratoderma blennorrhagica, painless oral ulcers, and circinate balanitis. A postdysenteric Reiter's syndrome can follow intestinal infection with *Shigella flexneri* or *Yersinea enterocolitica*.

     c. Psoriatic arthritis: about 7% of patients with psoriasis have an inflammatory arthritis. Psoriatic arthritis can be divided into five types:

       1. Arthritis of the distal interphalangeal joints.

TABLE 8-2.
Comparison of Seronegative Spondyloarthropathies*

Description	Ankylosing Spondylitis	Reiter's Syndrome	Psoriatic Arthropathy	Enteropathic Spondylitis
Sex	Men>Women	Men>Women	Women>Men	Women = Men
Age at onset	20	Any age	Any age	Any age
Uveitis	+	++	+	+
Conjunctivitis	-	+	-	-
Peripheral joints	Lower>Upper: often	Lower usually	Upper>Lower	Lower>Upper
Sacroiliitis	Always	Often	Often	Often
HLA-B27	95%	80%	20% (50% with-sacroiliitis)	50%
Enteropathy	+	+	+	?
Aortic regurgitation	+	+	?+	?
Familial aggregation	+	+	+	+
Risk for HLA-B27-positive individual	±20%	20%	?	?
Onset	Gradual	Sudden	Variable	Gradual
Urethritis	-	+	-	-
Skin involvement	-	+	++	-
Mucous membrane involvement	-	+	-	+
Symmetry (spinal)	+	-	-	+
Self-limiting	-	+/-	+/-	+/-
Remission, relapses	-	+/-	+/-	-

*Adapted from Calin A: The spondylarthropathies, in Wyngaarden JB, Smith LH (eds): Cecil Textbook of Medicine. Philadelphia, WB Saunders Co., 1985, p 1918. Used by permission.

       2. Symmetric polyarthritis resembling RA.
       3. Asymmetric oligoarthritis.
       4. Arthritis mutilans with severe involve-
          ment of the digits.
       5. Spondylitis: 50% of these patients will
          be HLA B27 positive.
    d. Enteropathic arthritides associated with in-
      flammatory bowel disease include:
       1. Large joint oligoarthritis.
       2. Spondylitis: 50% of these patients are
          HLA B27 positive.
F. Polymyalgia rheumatica (PMR). Presents in persons
   over 50 years old with severe myalgias, arthralgias,
   and stiffness in the pelvic girdle, shoulder girdle,
   and neck. Almost all patients will have Westergren
   sedimentation rates (ESRs) of over 40 mm/hour.
   Treatment with NSAIDs or low dose steroids is recommended.
G. Temporal arteritis (TA) (also known as giant cell arteritis).
    1. Presentation: generally presents in people over
      50 years old. Temporal arteritis can involve the
      temporal and ophthalmic arteries and other
      branches of the aortic arch. Disruption of artery
      walls and occlusion of affected arteries can oc-
      cur. In the ophthalmic artery, this can result in
      blindness, the most feared result of TA. Symp-
      toms of TA include temporal or occipital head-
      aches, masseter muscle pain with chewing, and
      visual abnormalities. Patients with TA are usu-
      ally over 50 years old and have Westergren
      ESRs of over 40 mm/hour. About 50% of pa-
      tients with TA also have PMR.
    2. Diagnosis: made by characteristic histologic
      findings including multinucleated giant cells on
      a temporal artery biopsy specimen.
    3. Treatment: initially with 40–60 mg prednisone
      daily.
H. Polymyositis (PM) and dermatomyositis (DM).
    1. Presentation: PM and DM are inflammatory
      skeletal muscle diseases that lead to proximal
      muscle weakness. DM is distinguished by a

dusky-red maculopapular rash over the dorsal PIP and MCP joints, the elbow, knees, medial malleoli, and face. Periorbital edema and a violaceous rash of the upper eyelids (heliotrope rash) are also characteristic. In adults with DM, an increased incidence of malignancies has been reported.

2. Classification: there are five groups of patients with PM/DM. Group 1: primary PM; Group 2: primary DM; Group 3: DM (or PM) associated with malignancy; Group 4: childhood DM (or PM) associated with vasculitis; Group 5: PM (or DM) associated with collagen-vascular disease.

3. Diagnosis: depends on the finding of elevated serum creatine phosphokinase (sCPK), evidence of myopathy on electromyography, and characteristic changes on a muscle biopsy specimen from a patient with proximal muscle weakness.

4. Treatment: corticosteroids and, in resistant cases, immunosuppressive or cytotoxic agents.

III. Vasculitides.
This group includes many diseases, only a few of which will be mentioned here.

A. Polyarteritis nodosum (PAN).
PAN typically afflicts middle-aged men. Pathologically there is involvement of small- and medium-sized muscular arteries. All layers of the arterial wall can be affected with inflammation and necrosis. Any organ can be affected but the arteries of the kidneys, the heart, the intestines, and the skin are most frequently involved. In addition to supportive measures, corticosteroids and immunosuppressive agents such as azathioprine and cyclophosphamide are used for treatment.

B. Churg-Strauss disease (allergic granulomatous angiitis).
This disease is characterized pathologically by a granulomatous vasculitis of small- and medium-

sized vessels. Patients generally have a long history
of asthma and present with a migratory pneumonitis. Other features include leukocytosis, peripheral
eosinophilia, and elevated IgE levels. Renal involvement is unusual.

C. Hypersensitivity vasculitis.
This group includes serum sickness, the vasculitis of
subacute bacterial endocarditis, vasculitis associated
with other connective tissue diseases, essential
mixed cryoglobulinemia, and can be associated with
malignancies.

D. Wegener's granulomatosis.
Characterized by a granulomatous vasculitis involving the upper and lower respiratory tracts and necrotizing glomerulonephritis.

E. Takayasu's arteritis (pulseless disease).
Characterized by involvement of the arteries arising
from the aortic arch with less frequent involvement
of the thoracic and abdominal aorta, pulmonary, and
renal arteries.

IV. Synovial fluid analysis (Table 8–3).

V. Radiologic clues to common arthropathies.

A. Osteoarthritis.
Joints affected by osteoarthritis are characterized by
subchrondral sclerosis and excess-bone proliferation
often called bone spurs. As articular cartilage is
lost, joint space narrowing will occur.

B. Rheumatoid arthritis.
Early on, periarticular osteopenia and soft tissue
swelling may be present. In more advanced disease,
joint space narrowing and bone erosions are present.
Erosions first develop near the attachments of the
joint capsules, commonly in the MCP, PIP, wrist,
and MTP joints.

C. Spondyloarthropathies.
The first radiologic sign of spondyloarthropathy is
usually sclerosis of the sacroiliac joints. Vertebral
changes include squaring of the vertebral bodies
early on, and then the formation of syndesmo-

TABLE 8–3.
Synovial Fluid Analysis*

Diagnosis	Appearance	Total White Cell Count per Cubic Millimeter†	Polymorphonuclear Cells	Mucin Clot Test	Synovial Fluid-Blood Glucose Difference (Mean Milligrams per Deciliter)	Miscellaneous (Crystals, Organisms)
Normal	Clear, pale yellow	0–200 (200)	<10%	Good	No significant difference‡	—
Group I (noninflammatory effusions)						
Degenerative joint disease; traumatic arthritis	Clear to slightly turbid	500–4000 (600)	<30%	Good	No significant difference	—
Group II (noninfectious, mildly inflammatory)						
Systemic lupus erythematosus; scleroderma	Clearly to slightly turbid	0–9000 (3000)	<20%	Good (occasionally fair)	No significant difference	Occasional LE cell; decreased complement

	Appearance	WBC/mm³	% PMN	Mucin clot	Glucose†	Special findings
Group III (Noninfectious severe inflammatory effusions)						
Gout	Turbid	100–160,000 (21,000)	~70%	Poor	10	Monosodium urate crystals
Pseudogout	Turbid	50–75,000 (14,000)	~70%	Fair-poor	Not enough data	Calcium pyrophosphate dihydrate crystals
Rheumatoid arthritis	Turbid	250–80,000 (19,000)	~70%	Poor	30	Decreased complement
Group IV (infectious inflammatory effusions)						
Acute bacterial	Very turbid	150–250,000 (80,000)	~90%	Poor	90	Culture positive for gram-positive or gram-negative bacteria
Tuberculosis	Turbid	2500–100,000 (20,000)	~60%	Poor	70	Culture positive for M. tuberculosis

*Adapted from Cohen AS: Specialized diagnostic procedures in rheumatic diseases, in Wyngaarden JB, Smith LH (eds): Cecil Textbook of Medicine. Philadelphia, WB Saunders Co, 1985, p 1907.
†Averages in parenthesis.
‡Less than 10 mg per deciliter difference.

phytes. Syndesmophytes are typically paravertebral ossifications. They can form all along the spinal column resulting in a bamboo spine appearance.

D. Gout.

The bone erosions of gout characteristically have an overhanging margin. The disease tends to be asymmetric. Tophi appear as nodular soft tissue swellings. They can calcify giving a radiographic appearance of a particulate soft tissue mass with a denser appearance than the surrounding soft tissue.

E. CPPD.

Chondrocalcinosis is frequently seen in CPPD. Fibrocartilage, especially in the menisci and in the triangular cartilage of the wrist, are frequently involved.

BIBLIOGRAPHY

Wyngaarden JB, Smith LH Jr (eds): *Cecil Textbook of Medicine,* ed 17. Philadelphia, WB Saunders Co, 1985, pp 1870–1904.
Kelly E: *Textbook of Rheumatology,* ed 2. Philadelphia, WB Saunders Co, 1985.

Allergy and Immunology

John Phelan, M.D.
San San Wong, M.D.
Nancy Lance, M.D.

I. Anaphylaxis.
  A. Definition: generalized IgE-mediated reaction requiring histamine and other vasoactive mediator release that may result in life-threatening symptoms.
  B. Anaphylactoid reactions: non IgE-mediated reactions causing symptoms indistinguishable from those of IgE-mediated anaphylaxis. Common examples are reactions to aspirin and nonsteroidal anti-inflammatory drugs, some intravenous antipyretics, opiates, and polymyxin B.
  C. Clinical manifestations of anaphylaxis (Table 9–1): The anaphylactic reactions usually occur immediately (within 20 to 30 minutes) after exposure to an antigen.
  D. Common causes of anaphylaxis:
    1. Antibiotics: penicillin, tetracycline, nitrofurantoin, streptomycin, and sulfonamides have been implicated. Penicillin is the prototypical drug-induced, IgE-mediated reaction. It is a hapten that binds to a host protein to become a complete antigen. More severe reactions occur with parenteral administration.
    2. Insect stings: bee, wasp, hornet, yellowjacket (most common). Systemic reactions occur in 0.5% to 5.0% of people who have been stung

TABLE 9–1.

Clinical Manifestations of Anaphylaxis*

System	Manifestation
Skin	Pruritus, flushing, erythema, angioedema, urticaria
Eye	Conjunctival suffusion, lacrimation, pruritus
Nose	Rhinorrhea, congestion, sneezing, pruritus
Upper airway	Oropharyngeal or laryngeal edema, hoarseness, stridor
Lower airway	Tachypnea, dyspnea, chest tightness, wheezing, use of accessory muscles of respiration, intercostal or sternal notch retractions, cyanosis
Cardiovascular	Tachycardia, irregular pulse, hypotension
Gastrointestinal	Nausea, vomiting, cramping, bloating, diarrhea (which may be bloody)
Neurologic	Fear of impending death, metallic taste, dizziness, syncope, perineal burning sensation, seizure, weakness

*Allergy and Immunology, Medical Knowledge Self-Assessment Program VII. 1986; p 91. Used by permission.

by *Hymenoptera*; however, fatal anaphylaxis is quite uncommon. Skin testing with venoms is the most sensitive technique for determining presence of venom-specific IgE antibody. The RAST test has a 15% false-negative rate.

3. Foods: commonly implicated are shellfish, peanuts, nuts, fish, and cottonseed.

4. Vaccines: pertussis, typhoid, and vaccines grown on egg embryo in patients sensitive to eggs.

5. Foreign protein agents: tetanus and diphtheria antitoxins, antilymphocyte globulin, and venom antitoxin.

6. Protein drugs: insulin, ACTH, estradiol, and vasopressin.

E. Therapy:

1. Initial therapy should be directed at supporting the circulatory system and maintaining an effec-

tive airway by giving oxygen, intravenous fluids, and aqueous epinephrine hydrochloride 1:1000 dilution 0.2–0.3 mg subcutaneously and repeating as necessary.

2. Patients receiving β-blockers may be refractory to standard anaphylaxis therapy. Glucagon infusion has on occasion been effective (2 U intravenously).

3. Administration of intravenous corticosteroids is recommended.

4. For severe bronchospasm, administration of the aerosol β-agonist aminophylline is indicated and mechanical ventilation may be necessary.

5. Late phase allergic responses can occur in 20% to 50% of patients and they should be observed and monitored for at least 8 to 12 hours in the hospital.

II. Radiologic contrast material anaphylactoid reaction.
  A. Scope of the problem:
    1. Occurs in 1% to 2% of all procedures.
    2. Similar to IgE-mediated hypersensitivity in that urticaria, angioedema, bronchospasm, and hypotension may occur.
    3. Vasomotor reactions including nausea, vomiting, flushing, and warmth occur in 5% to 8% of patients.
    3. A history of reaction is a predictive factor for recurrence in 17% to 35% of patients.
  B. Prophylaxis (modified from the Greenberger regimen):
    1. Prednisone 50 mg (or dose equivalent of other steroids) orally every 6 hours for three doses ending 1 hour prior to the procedure.
    2. Diphenhydramine 50 mg: intramuscularly 1 hour prior to the procedure.
    3. Document necessity of procedure and assure that no alternate imaging techniques are available.
    4. For emergency procedures:

      a. Hydrocortisone 200 mg intravenously stat and every 4 hours until the procedure is complete.

      b. Diphenhydramine 50 mg intramuscularly 1 hour prior to the procedure.

5. Outcome of prophylaxis:

      a. 92.5% of patients had no reaction.

      b. 7% had a minimal reaction such as pruritis or rhinorrhea requiring no intervention.

      c. Less than 1% will have anaphylaxis.

6. The benefit of the addition of cimetidine to the regimen is debatable.

7. For patients on long-term β-blockade, ephedrine 25 mg orally 1 hour prior to administration of contrast material has been effective in some situations (in addition to prednisone and diphenhydramine).

III. Penicillin (PCN) allergy skin testing and desensitization.

A. Penicillin hypersensitivity.

    1. Incidence: approximately 2% of patients.

      a. 2% to 13% of reactions have life-threatening manifestations that include: laryngeal edema (stridor), hypotension, bronchospasm, and cardiac arrhythmias.

    2. Skin testing for PCN hypersensitivity: Anaphylactic reactions correlate with positive skin test reactions to the minor breakdown products of PCN (e.g., penicilloate, penilloate) and PCN. Rare systemic reactions to the major determinant breakdown product have been reported. A major determinant mixture is commercially available (Pre pez) as standard PCN G. No minor determinant mixture is available.

      Skin testing begins by completing (prick) tests to the major and minor determinants and PCN G. Both negative and positive (histamine) controls are necessary for comparison. If scratch testing is negative, intradermal testing is conducted with the same antigens. If negative, the patient has less than 7% risk of immediate, potentially life-threatening reactions to penicillin. This does not preclude that delayed rashes, renal disease, etc. may be complications of therapy.

    3. Desensitization.

        a. Criteria/indications.

           i. Positive skin test.

          ii. No adequate alternative antibiotic may be substituted.

         iii. Life-threatening infection such that the risk and fatality from infection is greater than that of anaphylaxis.

        b. Procedures.

           i. Skin test.

          ii. Involvement of infectious disease and allergy consultants.

         iii. Formal consent.

         iv. Procedure performed in intensive care unit or controlled hospitalized setting.

          v. Epinephrine and benadryl as well as emergency equipment at the bedside.

         vi. Medical doctor present at all times.

IV. Immunologic tests.

    A. Acute phase reactants: multiple serum protein levels will be elevated during inflammation. Clinically measured acute phase reactants include: erythrocyte sedimentation rate (ESR), and C reactive protein (CRP). These reactants are elevated in response to nonspecific inflammation or tissue necrosis. CRP increases within hours, and decreases rapidly over days. ESR rises more slowly, peaks after several days, and may persist for weeks after inflammation has subsided.

    B. Rheumatoid factor (RF).

        1. Current chemical assays detect an IgM autoantibody directed against the CH2 domain of IgG.

        2. Methods.

           a. Latex agglutination: (positive test > 1:40).

Sensitive, but not specific for rheumatoid arthritis (RA). Latex beads coated with Ig.

   b. Sensitized sheep RBCs: (positive test > 1:20). Sheep RBC sensitized with anti-sheep antibody: specific but not sensitive for RA.

3. May be present in patients with RA in lower titers with systemic lupus erythematosus (SLE), chronic infectious diseases, malignancy, cryoglobulinemia, and chronic inflammatory disease.

C. Antinuclear antibodies (ANA).

   1. Four clinically significant patterns have been identified.

      a. Homogenous (diffuse): produced by the histone component of antideoxyribonucleoprotein (anti-DNP), is most frequently found in SLE, although seen with other collagen vascular diseases (particularly RA, Sjögrens syndrome, and in drug-induced lupus).

      b. Rim: produced by antibodies to double-stranded DNA. Is more specific for SLE although less frequent than the homogenous pattern.

      c. Nucleolar: caused by antibody to 4S-6S nucleolar RNA and is associated with scleroderma.

      d. Speckled: antibody to single stranded (denatured) DNA, extractable nuclear antigen (ENA), ribonucleoprotein (RNP), Smith antigen (SM), misc.

         i. High titers are associated with mixed connective tissue disease (MCTD); also positive in SLE, progressive systemic sclerosis (PSS), polymyositis, and RA.

         ii. May have extractable antibody to nuclear antigens: anti-Smith is specific for SLE but has provided only 30% sensitivity; anti-RNP is most commonly detected in SLE, also positive in MCTD in high titers, PSS, polymyositis, and RA; anti-SSA is present in Sjögrens syndrome and seronegative SLE (35% prevalence); anti-SSB is strongly associated with Sjögrens syndrome although may be detected in SLE (15% prevalence).

2. Drug induced lupus most frequently produces a homogenous pattern, but one can also see a speckled pattern. Drugs most often implicated include procainamide, hydralazine, and isoniazid.

3. Positive ANA is also seen with cirrhosis, ulcerative colitis, infectious mononucleosis, chronic active hepatitis (CAH), chronic lymphocytic leukemia (CLL), and acute lymphocytic leukemia (ALL).

4. Anti-smooth muscle antibody is highly specific for primary biliary cirrhosis (PBC); can also be seen with CAH and viral hepatitis.

D. Circulating immune complex (CIC) detection: No single CIC assay is entirely adequate, therefore, two assays are necessary.

1. Raji cell assay is a lymphoblastoid cell with B lymphocyte characteristics. Has low affinity FC receptors on the cell surface for binding immunoglobulin and a high affinity for binding complement components C3bi, and C3d (CR2 receptor).

2. C1q binding assay is the first component of the complement cascade to recognize antigen-antibody (Ag-Ab) complexes. Currently C1q is bound in a solid phase; the patient's serum is added and if immune complexes of IgG or IgM are present, they bind to the C1q. The bound immune complex is detected with a radioisotope- or enzyme-labeled anti-immunoglobulin.

E. Complement (Fig 9–1).

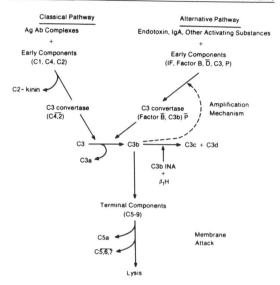

FIG 9–1

Diagram of the classic and alternative complement pathways. These two pathways converge at C3 to form a common terminal pathway that results in cell lysis. Cleavage of complement components produces biologically active fragments. (From Gilliland BC: Introduction to clinical immunology, in Harrison, Petersdorf, Adams, et al (eds): *Principles of Internal Medicine*, ed 10. New York, McGraw Hill Book Co, 1983, p 351. Used by permission.)

Individual complement components or the integrity of the entire pathway are measured. C3, C4, factor B, and properdin are measured with an immunodiffusion test.

1. Abnormal levels of C3 may be detected when either the alternate or classical pathways have been activated.

    2. Decreased C4 and C1q levels suggest classical pathway activity.

    3. Decreased factor B and properdin levels suggest alternative pathway activity.

    4. CH50: photometric test quantifying hemolytic activity of the entire complement system; it is a functional assay that suggests complement deficiency when no lysis is detected. A complement consumption test is performed when reduced levels are quantitated.

  F. Complement deficiencies.

    1. C1R, C1S: SLE-like syndrome.

    2. C2: SLE, dermatomyositis, vasculitis, glomerulonephritis.

    3. C3: recurrent bacterial infection, SLE.

    4. C4, C5: SLE-like syndrome, *Neisseria* meningitis, disseminated gonococcal infection.

    5. C5 dysfunction: recurrent infection with gram-negative bacteria and eczema (Lenier's syndrome).

    6. C6: *Neisseria* meningitis.

    7. C7: *Neisseria* meningitis.

    8. C8: *Neisseria* meningitis, disseminated gonococcal infection.

    9. C1 esterase deficiency: hereditary angioedema.

V. Coombs type III disease (immune complex).

  A. Causes.

    1. Use of heterologous serum.

    2. Medications: PCN, sulfa, and dilantin are the most common.

  B. Clinical syndrome occurs within 7 to 14 days after antigen stimulation: fever, malaise, arthralgias (affecting large joints), nausea, lymphadenopathy (usually cervical), a morbilliform rash (begins periumbilical spreading to trunk), or a petechial rash most frequently on the lower extremities (leukocytoclastic vasculitis).

  C. Pathogenesis: These foreign antigens initiate antibody formation and circulating immune complexes may be deposited in a variety of organ systems. The process is self limiting and 10% to 20% of patients show slow elimination of the immune complexes.

D. Diagnosis: appropriate clinical presentation. Serologically: elevated circulating immune complexes C1Q; Raji cell: decreased C3, decreased C4, and decreased CH50 may be seen.

E. Treatment: removal of antigen. If the disease requires therapy, then steroids are helpful for controlling the inflammatory state (prednisone 1 mg/kg/day orally for 7 to 14 days with a rapid taper).

VI. Primary immunodeficiency states (Table 9–2).

VII. Cryoimmunoglobulins.

Cryoglobulins are immunoglobulins, which at low temperatures (4°C) spontaneously precipitate and resolubilize when the temperature is raised (37°C). Fibronectin is another example of protein that is cryoprecipitable.

Collection of cryoglobulins: blood is drawn and kept warm at 37°C for 4 hours, clotted, and separated by centrifugation at 37°C. Serum is stored at 4°C for 5 days. Cryoprecipitate is then washed several times and resuspended at 37°C. Cryoglobulin concentration is measured by centrifugation at 4°C in a hematocrit tube to determine the relative amount of cryoglobulin (cryocrit). Alternately, the cryoglobulin is resolubilized and quantitated compared with an albumin control (Lowry). These cryoglobulins may be separated with gel filtration and purified.

A. Types of cryoglobulins.

1. Type I: monoclonal cryoglobulinemia IgM, IgG, IgA or Bence-Jones protein. Diseases associated with B-cell or plasma cell derived malignancies (e.g., multiple myeloma, lymphoma, and Waldenström's macroglobulinemia).

2. Type II: mixed cryoglobulinemia is associated with a monoclonal immunoglobulin (Ig) directed against IgG (i.e., IgM-IgG, IgA-IgG, IgG-IgG). Diseases associated with this type include lymphoproliferative disorders, myeloproliferative states, and inflammatory disease (SLE). May have rheumatoid factor activity.

3. Type III: mixed polyclonal cryoglobulins consist of more than one class of polyclonal immunoglobulins. This is the most common type of cryoglobulin. May have rheumatoid factor activity.

Diseases associated with this type include:
   a. Connective tissue disease: SLE, RA, polyarteritis nodosa, ankylosing spondylitis, and Sjögrens Syndrome.
   b. Infectious agents: Subacute bacterial endocarditis, post-streptococcal nephritis, cytomegalovirus mononucleosis, syphillis, toxoplasmosis, infectious mononucleosis, echinococcosis, lyme disease, and chronic hepatitis B.
   c. Other chronic diseases: sarcoidosis, intestinal bypass arthritis, ulcerative colitis, celiac disease, chronic liver disease, and cutaneous plasmacytosis.

4. Essential cryoglobulinemia: cryoglobulins are detected without evidence of another systemic disease. Essential cryoglobulinemia may be seen with types I or II, but is usually type III.

B. Clinical manifestations.

Patients with type I monoclonal cryoglobulinemia usually present with symptoms suggestive of hyperviscosity, which include headaches, lethargy, bleeding, visual difficulties, Raynaud's phenomenon, fingertip necrosis, distal gangrene and ulceration, and thrombosis.

Patients with type II and III mixed cryoglobulinemia usually have symptoms similar to immune complex diseases (i.e., cutaneous and systemic vasculitis, glomerulonephritis). Cutaneous manifestations are the most common findings and include vascular purpura, acute necrotizing vasculitis, and urticarial-like lesions. The second most common symptom is arthralgia with erythema and joint destruction. Neurologic symptoms include peripheral neuropathy; central nervous system involvement is

TABLE 9–2.
Primary Immunodeficiency States‡

Designation	Phenotypic Expression	Pathogenesis	Inheritance	Clinical Manifestations
Severe combined immunodeficiency (SCID)	Decreased CMI*, Ab†, ascending T-cell, B-cell, +/− decreased phagocytes	Hematopoietic stem cell deficiency	Autosomal recessive occasional sporadic x-linked	Disseminated pyogenic, fungal, viral infection in first weeks of life
DiGeorge's syndrome	Decreased CMI*, Ab†, decreased T-cell	Thymic hypoplasia	Nonfamilial	Disseminated infection, hypoparathyroid, other birth defects
Ataxia telangiectasia	Decreased CMI*, T-cell, partial decreased Ab†, IgA (40%)	Abnormal differentiation of B, T-cells	Autosomal recessive	Disseminated infection, cerebellar ataxia, telangiectasia, ovarian dysgenesis (↓ alpha fetoprotein)
Thymoma	Decreased Ab†, pre-B, B +/−, decreased CMI*	Unknown effect on hematopoiesis	None	Disseminated infection, eosinophilopenia, aplastic anemia, pure red cell aplasia
X-linked hypogam-maglobulinemia	Decreased Ab†, B-cell	Pre B-cell deficiency	X-linked	Persistent pyogenic infections particularly respiratory tract, ears, conjuctivae

Selective IgA deficiency	Decreased IgA, +/− decreased T-cell	Abnormal terminal differentiation B-cell	Recessive, dominant	Diarrhea, *Giardia*, recurrent sinusitis, bronchiectasis, uveitis, atopy, eczema, most are asymptomatic
IgG deficiencies	Decreased Ab†, sometimes only to specific antigen	B-cell defect	Sporatic recessive, X-linked	Persistant pyogenic infection particularly respiratory tract
Wiskott-Aldrich syndrome	Decreased Ab† to some antigens, decreased phagocytes, T, B-cell (IgM, IgA, IgE)	Possible decreased lymphocyte-derived chemotactic factor	X-linked	Otitis media, pyogenic infection, hemorrhage of petechiae, (thrombocytopenia)
Common variable immunodeficiency (CVID)	Decreased Ab†, CMI* +/− decreased B, T-cell	Intrinsic T/B cell defect	Episodic or familial	Respiratory infection, diarrhea
Terminal complement deficiency	Decreased C5, C6,C7, or C8	Decreased complement-mediated killing	Autosomal recessive	*Neisseria* infections
Primary phagocytic defects	Decreased bacterial killing or decreased motility	Decreased peroxide or superoxide production or decreased motility	Unknown, recessive, X-linked	Pyogenic or fungal infection

*CMI = Cell-Mediated immunity.
†A6 = antibody.
*Adapted from Stein JH: *Internal Medicine*, ed 2. Boston, Little Brown & Co, 1987, pp 1226–1227. Used by permission.

rare and usually secondary to arterial involvement.
The hyperviscosity syndrome is rare.

C. Treatment.

In type I associated with the hyperviscosity syndrome, plasmapheresis is the mainstay of therapy.
In patients with type II or III with circulating immune complex disorders, treatment includes steroids
and cytotoxic agents (i.e., cyclophosphamide). In
secondary cases, the underlying systemic illness
should be treated.

VIII. Urticaria.

A. Definition:

1. Urticaria is characterized by pruritic, raised,
   circumscribed skin lesions with erythema and
   edema involving superficial portions of the dermis. These lesions vary in size from 1–2 mm
   to several centimeters, usually multiple with
   each lesion persisting less than 24 hours. On
   resolution, there is no hyperpigmentation at the
   site of the hive.

2. Acute urticaria: symptoms last less than 6
   weeks, the cause is often readily apparent, and
   there is an increased incidence in atopic patients.

3. Chronic urticaria: symptoms last longer than 6
   weeks, occurs at any age, women are more
   commonly affected than men, and the majority
   of cases are idiopathic; however, the cause may
   be identified in 5% to 20% of patients.
   General occurrence: 20% of population.

B. Pathophysiology and etiology:

1. Allergen-induced, IgE-mediated mediator release can account for many cases of acute urticaria, but the role of IgE in chronic urticaria is
   debatable.

2. Medications such as PCN and sulfas are the
   prototype for causing acute urticaria. Aspirin
   ingestion can produce exacerbations of chronic
   urticaria in 40% of patients; however, the

mechanism is generally nonimmunologic and is due to effects on arachidonic acid metabolism.

3. Foods such as seafood, fish, nuts, peanuts, and eggs are commonly implicated in the cause of acute urticaria, much less often the cause of chronic urticaria. Food additives such as tartrazine, a yellow dye; azo dyes; benzoates; and salicylates are also implicated as a cause of acute and chronic urticaria.

4. Insect bites and aero-allergens may produce urticaria in sensitized patients. Urticaria secondary to the latter is routinely associated with nasal or ocular symptoms.

5. Immune-complex-mediated activation of the serum complement cascade can cause increased vascular permeability by release of the anaphylotoxins C3a and C5a, which in turn release histamine from cutaneous mast cells. Examples in which complement-mediated histamine releases may be a factor in the pathogenesis of urticaria include cryoglobulinemia, the leukocytoclastic vasculitis of the hypocomplementemic urticaria-vasculitis syndrome, hepatitis B prodromal reaction, and some blood transfusion reactions.

6. Infectious causes include hepatitis B, parasitic infections, and rarely infectious mononucleosis, which may precipitate urticaria. Drugs such as polymyxin B, morphine, and its derivatives are capable of inducing direct release of histamine from basophils.

7. Urticaria may be categorized according to some blood-based causative factors: ingestants, contactants, aero-allergins, physical stimuli, and systemic diseases. Some more commonly recognized forms of urticaria include the following:

   a. Pressure urticaria: unknown etiology; constant pressure of 4 to 6 hours applied to the skin in sensitized individuals may cause erythematous deep local swelling; common sites are palms, soles, and buttocks or in areas of tight garments; histologically, the lesion is surrounded by infiltration of mononuclear cells with or without eosinophils, no evidence of immunoglobulins or complement with immunofluorescent staining; it is often refractory to antihistamine, and corticosteroid therapy may be needed.

b. Dermographism occurs in 2.5% of the population. Gentle stroking of the skin causes linear wheels. A secondary form of dermographism occurs in cutaneous mastocytosis.

c. Cold-induced urticaria is characterized by an acute onset of urticaria within minutes of exposure to cold. Cold water swimming can cause anaphylaxis. Mast cell mediator release is the possible mechanism. Screen with the ice cube test (application of ice cubes to the skin for 4 to 5 minutes with resultant 4 mm prutitic wheal as skin rewarms in 5 to 15 minutes is a positive test). The drug of choice is cyproheptadine. Secondary forms of cold urticaria are associated with cryoglobulinemia, cryofibrinogenemia, cold agglutinin disease, and paroxysmal cold hemoglobinemia. Secondary forms have a negative ice cube test.

d. Solar urticaria: Solar-induced reactions are divided into six categories depending on the wavelength that induces the cutaneous response. Brief (minutes) exposure to light or sun causes erythematous pruritic wheals in two types of solar reactions that may be passively transferred by serum to a nonreactive control (P-K reaction). Genetic forms are seen in genetic abnormalities of protoporphyrin IX metabolism.

e. Cholinergic urticaria is characterized by small punctate urticaria surrounded by an erythematous flare associated with severe pruritis. It is associated with hot showers, exercise, emotional tensions or episodes of fever. Increased plasma histamine has been observed during these reactions. This urticaria responds to hydroxyzine hydrochloride.

f. Exercise-induced anaphylactic syndrome is usually seen in runners or occurs with prolonged strenuous exercise. Symptoms usually begin about 30 minutes after exercise is started and can present with various combinations of symptoms: urticaria with or without angioedema, respiratory distress, or hypotension. Cutaneous mast cell degranulation has been implicated in the pathogenesis. In some patients, this syndrome of attack is preceded by ingestion of specific food such as shellfish or celery.

C. Evaluation of urticaria:

A thorough history and physical examination to rule out any evidence of systemic disease is important. General screening should include CBC, Westergren sedimentation rate, urinalysis, SMA-12, thyroid battery, and hepatitis screen.

In patients in whom you suspect vasculitis or complement related causes of urticaria, an autoimmune profile and possible skin biopsy should be done.

For physical urticaria, simple tests such as the ice cube test, local heat application, and gentle stroking of the skin can be done to bring on urticaria. For potential secondary causes of cold urticaria; cryoglobulins and an RPR should be obtained.

IX. Angioedema.

Is an asymmetric swelling primarily in the subcutaneous tissue, rarely pruritic, involving leakage from postcapillary venules. It may involve any part of the body as single or multiple lesions. The lesions may last a few hours or up to 3 days. Characteristic locations are periorbital areas, lip, and genital areas. Trunk, extremities, tongue, pharynx, and viscera can also be involved. It can be a manifestation of anaphylactic reactions to drugs, insect stings, foods, or other allergens.

A. Hereditary angioedema (HAE).

Clinically presents as self-limited recurrent attacks of angioedema involving the GI tract, upper respiratory tract, and skin. Soft tissue trauma can be a trigger to the development of the attacks (e.g., tooth extraction may trigger development of laryngeal edema and airway obstruction). GI involvement often causes abdominal pain, nausea, and vomiting. Onset is usually in children or young adults. It is autosomal dominant; however, family history may be vague. Eight to five percent of patients have low levels of an antigenically normal and functionally normal C1 inhibitor protein (type I). The remainder of patients have normal or elevated levels of nonfunctional C1 inhibitor protein (type II). C4 is decreased between attacks and nearly absent during an attack. Possible mechanisms: C1 inhibitor protein stabilizes the C1qrs complex. In the absence of this protein, C1r is autoactivated and leads to subsequent activation of the classical pathway resulting in low C4 and C2. C1 inhibitor protein is also the inhibitor of both kallikrein system and activated Hageman factor resulting in bradykinin release, which may be a factor in causing the edema. Treatment: anabolic agents such as danazol and stanozolol have been used. They enhance the C1 inhibitor protein synthesis. Epinephrine, corticosteroids, and β-agonists have not been effective in the treatment of HAE.

B. Acquired C1 inhibitor protein deficiency.

Is associated with B cell lymphoproliferative disorders predominantly or connective tissue diseases such as SLE. Clinically, they are identical to HAE, although the pattern is sporadic, not autosomal.

Low C1, C1q, C4, C2, C1 inhibitor protein levels
are present. C1 inhibitor deficiency is due to either
autoantibodies to C1 inhibitor or antiidiotypic antibodies leading to increased turnover of C1 inhibitor.
Treatment requires the treatment of the underlying
disease. Although attentuated androgens have been
used, they have not been successful.

X. Antihistamines.

When one cannot find a cause or if the precipitating
agent cannot be avoided, symptomatic treatment can be
attained with antihistamines.

A. H1 type.

The mainstay of therapy for urticaria. Multiple H1
blockers are available and each may be effective if
an appropriate dose is administered. The side effect
of potentially profound lethargy is a limiting factor.
New nonsedating H1 blockers (e.g., terfenadine) at
larger doses than routinely prescribed for rhinitis are
effective as are some of the tricyclic antidepressants
(e.g., doxepin hydrochloride).

1. Hydroxyzine: it has antihistamine, anticholi-
   nergic, and antiserotonic effects. It is the most
   potent drug in suppressing chronic urticaria and
   it is the drug of choice for cholinergic urticaria.
2. Cyproheptadine hydrochloride: drug of choice
   for cold urticaria.

B. H2 blockers: cimetidine or ranitidine. The additive
effect of these agents is debatable.

C. Corticosteroids: effective for the treatment of de-
layed-pressure urticaria and severe serum sickness
type reaction that fails to respond to other medications.

BIBLIOGRAPHY

Allergy/Immunology

Greenberger PA, et al: Prophylaxis against repeated radiocontrast media reactions in 85 cases. *Arch Intern Med* 1985;
145:297–320.
Greenberger PA, et al: Pretreatment of high risk patients re-

quiring radiocontrast media studies. *J Allergy Clin Immunol* 1981; 67:185–187.

Kaplan AP, et al: Allergic skin disorders. *JAMA* 1987; 258:2905–2909.

Matthews KP: Urticaria and angioedema. *J Allergy Clin Immunol* 1983; 72:1–14.

Patterson R: Urticaria, angioedema, and idiopathic anaphylaxis, in *Allergies, Diseases, Diagnosis and Management*, ed 3. Philadelphia, JB Lippincott Co, 1985, pp 440–458.

Coffey FL, Zile MR, Luskin AT: Immunologic tests of value in diagnosis: part 2. *Postgrad Med* 1981; 70:183–187.

Lint TF: Laboratory detection of complement activation and complement deficiencies. *Am Soc Med Tech* 1982; 48:743–748.

Luskin AT, et al: Clinical and laboratory evaluation of immunologic disease. *Compr Ther* 1985; 11:27–37.

Kelly E: *Textbook of Rheumatology*, ed 2. Philadelphia, WB Saunders Co, 1985, 1344–1349.

Endocrinology

David Baldwin, Jr., M.D.
Daniel Hirsch, M.D.
James Lane, M.D.

DIABETES MELLITUS

I. Type I Diabetes Mellitus

A. Etiology.

Most cases of diabetes mellitus are diagnosed within the first three decades of life; however, it may occur at any age. An abrupt onset of polyuria and polydipsia is common. Patients are prone to ketosis and ketoacidosis. This disease is caused by chronic autoimmune destruction of the insulin-producing β cells. HLA antigens, DR3, and DR4 are genetic markers for susceptibility to this disease. The risk of developing the disease by a first degree relative of a type I diabetic is 1:20.

B. Treatment.

All patients with type I diabetes require immediate insulin therapy. The goal of insulin therapy in type I diabetes is to approximate normoglycemia without incurring unacceptable levels of hypoglycemia. All patients should perform home blood glucose monitoring two to four times each day. Urine glucose testing correlates poorly with actual blood glucose measurements. Daily home blood glucose monitoring data should be supplemented by the performance of glycohemoglobin testing. This test integrates the mean level of glycemia over the previous 2 to 3 months and gives an overall measure of diabetic control. There are essentially two approaches to insulin therapy in the type I diabetic (Table 10–1).

TABLE 10–1.
Therapeutic Insulins

Type	Onset	Peak	Duration
Regular intravenous	5 min	20 min	40 min
Regular intramuscular	30 min	60 min	90 min
Regular subcutaneous	60 min	3 hr	6 hr
NPH subcutaneous	4 hr	6–8 hr	10–16 hr
Lente subcutaneous	4 hr	6–8 hr	10–16 hr
Ultralente subcutaneous	8–12 hr	12–18 hr	18–28 hr

The first is to give an injection of the intermediate-acting insulin NPH mixed with short-acting regular insulin each morning before breakfast and repeated each evening before supper. Lente, the other intermediate-acting insulin, is not recommended because much of the rapid action of regular insulin is lost when it is mixed with Lente insulin. The dose of regular insulin is adjusted according to the blood sugar level 4 hours later. The dose of NPH insulin is adjusted according to the blood sugar level 8 to 12 hours later. An alternate approach is to deliver a continuous basal level of insulin supplemented by a bolus of insulin with each meal. The basal insulin can be given by continuous infusion of regular insulin by a portable pump, or by a single daily subcutaneous injection of ultralente insulin. The patient also takes additional regular insulin with each meal. The doses of regular insulin are adjusted according to blood glucose values obtained 3 to 4 hours later. The rate of basal infusion by pump or the dose of ultralente is determined by the morning fasting blood glucose level. Patients should be taught to vary the dose of their regular insulin before each meal according to an individualized algorithm based on blood glucose readings. During intercurrent illness, more frequent blood glucose monitoring as well as urine ketone monitoring is required. Fasting blood glucose values between 80 and 120 and postprandial blood glucose values between 100 and 160 are the goals of excellent diabetic control.

C. Diabetic ketoacidosis.

This is a decompensated state consisting of severe hyperglycemia, dehyration, and ketone body formation with acidosis. It is caused usually by poor compliance with insulin therapy or by superimposed infection. The initial evaluation consists of a fingerstick blood glucose measurement and a rapid physical examination. Attention is given to potential sites of infection such as meningitis, sinusitis, pyelonephritis, and pneumonia. Blood is sent for chemistries, pH, acetone measurement, complete blood count, and cultures. Therapy consists of intravenous fluids and insulin. In young patients, rehydration can generally be vigorous, 0.9% NaCl given at 500 mL per hour for the first 2 L, provided they have normal cardiac and renal function. After that, 0.45% NaCl may be given at 100–200 mL/hr depending on clinical assessment. Initial serum potassium measurements may be low, normal, or high. Potassium replacement should begin once the serum potassium is less than 4.0 mEq/L. Most patients will eventually require 100–200 mEq of potassium chloride. Serum electrolytes generally should be checked every 2 hours. Ketones should be checked every 4 hours. Insulin should be given via a continuous intravenous infusion of regular insulin at 0.1 U/kg/hr. Ten to fifteen units of intravenous regular insulin may be given as an initial loading bolus. Blood glucose levels should be tested with a fingerstick every hour. When the blood glucose level reaches 250, the insulin infusion rate may be decreased to 0.05–0.075 U/kg/hr. At that time, 5% dextrose should be added to the intravenous fluid (D5.45% NaCl with supplemental potassium). The rate should be adjusted to keep the blood glucose level between 150 and 250 while further insulin and hydration promote clearing of ketones. The insulin infusion should continue until urine ketones are di-

minishing and serum bicarbonate measurements
have returned to normal. At that point, the patient
may be switched to an injection of subcutaneous
regular insulin every 6 hours or preferably to a subcutaneous injection of an NPH and regular mixture
every 12 hours. The intravenous insulin infusion
must not be turned off until 2 to 3 hours after the
first subcutaneous injection of regular insulin. Frequent blood glucose measurements by finger-sticks
should continue every 3 to 6 hours as the doses of
subcutaneous insulin are adjusted. Studies in typical, young, type I diabetic patients with ketoacidosis
have shown that supplemental intravenous bicarbonate or phosphate is unnecessary. *Infection must be
aggressively sought and treated with appropriate
emperic antibiotics.*

II. Type II Diabetes.

    A. Etiology.

        Type II diabetes usually occurs in the fourth to sev-
enth decades. There is often a strong family history.
Most patients are overweight. Rarely, type II diabetes may occur in patients in their 20s or 30s. The
disease is caused by insulin resistance associated
with obesity and by a relative defect in insulin secretion. Type II diabetes can generally be diagnosed
by several fasting glucose measurements greater
than 150 or by several postprandial glucose measurements greater than 200, or by a significantly elevated glycohemoglobin measurement. Oral glucose
tolerance testing is generally considered unnecessary.

    B. Therapy.

        A balanced low calorie diet aimed at weight loss is
the cornerstone of therapy of type II diabetes. Most
patients who require pharmacologic therapy can be
treated with one of the oral agents. In general, one
of the newer agents such as Glipizide or Glyburide
is preferred. Since 80% of type II diabetics will respond to oral agents satisfactorally, all type II diabetics without urine ketones at the time of

presentation deserve a trial of oral agents. Some patients however, may require insulin therapy. NPH or NPH and regular insulin each morning will often give adequate diabetic control. Occasionally, patients need twice a day NPH or twice a day NPH and regular insulin. All therapeutic options in type II diabetes are best guided with home blood glucose monitoring data, and serial measurement of glycohemoglobin.

C. Hyperosmolar nonketotic coma.

This severe decompensation of type II diabetes usually occurs in elderly patients and has a mortality rate of 10% to 30%. Patients are usually severely dehydrated. The precipitating cause is infection in 50% of cases and is iatrogenic in 25% of cases secondary to insulin withdrawal, steroids, or thiazide diuretics. Treatment is quite similar to that of diabetic ketoacidosis and consists of judicious intravenous rehydration, continuous intravenous insulin infusion, and aggressive diagnosis and treatment of underlying infection.

HYPOGLYCEMIA

I. Signs and symptoms.

There are two types of hypoglycemic signs and symptoms: adrenergic and neuroglycopenic. The adrenergic type consists of tachycardia, sweating, tremor, and irritability; whereas neuroglycopenic symptoms consist of headache, blurred vision, confusion, seizures, and coma. Patients with autonomic neuropathy or patients who are taking β-blocking drugs may have blunted or absent adrenergic warning symptoms.

II. Etiology.

Most true hypoglycemia in adults occurs in the fasting stage. Rarely, postprandial reactive hypoglycemia may occur, usually in patients who have undergone previous gastric surgery (the dumping syndrome) or in occasional patients with an insulinoma. Drugs are a common cause of fasting hypoglycemia. They include insulin, sulfylu-

reas, salicylates, pentamidine, quinine, and ethanol.
Fasting hypoglycemia may occur in endstage liver failure, endstage kidney failure, adrenal insufficiency, panhypopituitarism, and sepsis. Although β-cell tumors of
the pancreas (insulinoma) are rare, they are an important
cause of fasting hypoglycemia. Additionally, large retroperitoneal sarcomas have also been associated with fasting hypoglycemia. Hypothermia and hypoglycemia
commonly occur together, especially in alcoholics.

III. Diagnosis.
Most cases of fasting hypoglycemia can be correctly diagnosed with a prolonged fast. Blood glucose levels are
monitored every 2 to 4 hours for up to 72 hours. Most
patients with true fasting hypoglycemia will develop
symptoms of neuroglycopenia in association with blood
glucose values less than 40. At the time of hypoglycemia, samples of serum and plasma must be obtained for
measurement of insulin and c-peptide. Patients taking
sulfylureas or patients with an insulinoma will have elevated levels. Other causes for fasting hypoglycemia such
as retroperitoneal tumors, adrenal insufficiency, renal
failure, or sepsis will invariably have low, suppressed
insulin and C-peptide levels. Serum proinsulin levels
may be useful in diagnosing insulinoma. The vast majority of cases of fasting hypoglycemia can be correctly diagnosed with this approach.

IV. Treatment.
Most patients who have drug-induced hypoglycemia will
recover with supportive intravenous glucose and time to
allow the drug to be cleared from the circulation. 50%
dextrose is given as a bolus followed by 10% dextrose
infusion with frequent finger-stick blood glucose monitoring. Underlying causes such as sepsis or adrenal insufficiency must be sought.

THYROID DISEASE

    I. Hyperthyroidism.
       A. Signs and symptoms.

    1. Anxiety.

    2. Fine tremor.

    3. Moist skin.

    4. Tachycardia.

    5. Atrial fibrillation.

    6. Proximal muscle weakness.

    7. Diarrhea.

    8. Stare and lid lag.

    9. Fatigue.

    10. Weight loss.

Weight loss and/or atrial fibrillation are often the only clues in elderly patients.

B. Etiology.

    1. Graves' disease (80%).

    Graves' disease is an autoimmune disease in which thyroid stimulating immunoglobulins are produced and bind to the thyroid stimulating hormone (TSH) receptor on the thyroid, causing hyperthyroidism. Many patients have exophthalmos and/or a thyroid bruit.

    2. Toxic multinodular goiter usually occurs in elderly patients.

    3. Toxic uninodular goiter (usually an adenoma).

    4. Subacute thyroiditis.

    This may be either the silent lymphocytic type or the tender granulomatous type. These may occur spontaneously or after pregnancy. A discharge of stored thyroid hormone causes hyperthyroidism for 1 to 2 months followed by a transient hypothyroidism and a return of euthyroidism. Granulomatous thyroiditis is marked by an extremely elevated westergren sedimentation rate.

    5. Exogenous thyroid hormone intake (iatrogenic or factitious).

    6. Iodine-induced hyperthyroidism.

    7. TSH-secreting pituitary adenoma (very rare).

C. Evaluation.

Measurement of serum T4, T3 RU, free thyroxine index (FTI), and TSH is necessary. Pregnant patients, patients taking estrogen preparations, or patients with chronic hepatitis may have an elevated total T4 but the free thyroxin index should be normal. All true cases of hyperthyroidism should be marked by an abnormally suppressed TSH with the exception of the very rare instance of a TSH-secreting pituitary adenoma. Some patients with the sick euthyroid syndrome may have hyperthyroxinemia but TSH as measured with ultrasensitive techniques should be normal and not suppressed. An I-123 scan and 24-hour uptake test should be performed next. The thyroid scan will facilitate diagnosis of nodular thyroid disease. The I-123 24-hour uptake (normal range 15% to 30%) test is usually strikingly elevated in Graves' disease. The 24-hour uptake test may be in the upper range of normal or elevated in nodular thyroid disease. The uptake is extremely low (less than 5%) in iodine-induced hyperthyroidism, subacute thyroiditis, and exogenous thyroid hormone ingestion.

D. Treatment.

Younger patients with Graves' disease who have had thyrotoxicosis for a short time and who have a small goiter have a 20% to 30% chance of a lasting complete remission of the disease after 9 to 12 months of antithyroid drug therapy. Propylthiouracil (50–150 mg orally every 8 hours) inhibits organification within the thyroid and inhibits peripheral T4 to T3 conversion. Methimazole (5–40 mg/day) only inhibits intrathyroidal organification. These drugs work slowly, and results are generally not seen until after 5 to 10 days of therapy. Side effects include skin rash (10%) and neutropenia (occurring less than 1% of the time). Alternate therapeutic options include radioactive I-131 and subtotal thyroidectomy. Radioactive iodine is generally not used in children, and subtotal thyroidectomy is generally not used in elderly patients. It takes between 2 to 6 months to see the full effect of radioactive iodine treatment. Occasionally, second and third doses are required for complete control of hyperthyroidism. There is a 50% to 90% chance of late hypothyroidism developing after radioactive iodine therapy.

E. Thyroid storm.

Thyroid storm is a medical emergency usually triggered by superimposed acute stress, such as infection. Patients have high fever, severe agitation, psychosis, severe tachycardia, atrial fibrillation, and often have nausea, vomiting, and dehydration. Treatment consists of large doses of propylthiouracil (150–250 mg every 8 hours). Iodide (SSKI, four to eight drops in water four times a day) is given to inhibit thyroid hormone release. Intravenous fluids are given, and intravenous or oral propranolol is used to control tachycardia. Hydrocortisone 50–75 mg intravenously every 6 hours is usually included. An underlying infection or other acute medical illness must be aggressively diagnosed and treated.

II. Hypothyroidism.

A. Signs and symptoms.

The signs and symptoms may be subtle, especially in elderly patients. They include fatigue, depression, lethargy and mental status change, bradycardia, constipation, dry skin, alopecia, hypothermia, prolonged relaxation of the deep tendon reflexes, and nonpitting edema.

B. Etiology.

1. Primary hypothyroidism.

The most common cause of primary hypothyroidism is autoimmune destruction of the thyroid by Hashimoto's disease. This is a common entity occurring in 2% to 4% of all patients over 60 years old. Antimicrosomal and antithyroglobulin antibodies are present in the serum of 90% of these patients. Thyroidectomy and radioactive I-131 therapy are other important causes of primary hypothyroidism. Additionally, drugs such as propylthiouracil, and Methimizole, lithium, iodine, and amiodarone may

also inhibit thyroid function and cause primary
hypothyroidism.

  2. Secondary hypothyroidism.

A variety of destructive processes of the pituitary gland and hypothalamus may cause secondary hypothyroidism and these are discussed
in the section on panhypopituitarism.

C. Diagnosis.

  1. Routine laboratory testing.

There are many nonspecific abnormalities seen
on routine laboratory tests of patients with hypothyroidism. They include a normocytic or
macrocytic anemia, and an elevated creatinine
phosphokinase (CPK), serum glutamic oxaloacetic transaminase (SGOT), lactate dehydrogenase (LDH), or cholesterol level. Hyponatremia
may also occasionally be seen. Patients with
hypothyroidism may also present with transuda-
tive effusions.

  2. Thyroid function testing.

Serum T4, free thyroxin index (FTI), and TSH.
If the FTI is low and the TSH is elevated, this
is consistent with the diagnosis of primary hypothyroidism and replacement therapy can be
initiated. However, if both the T4 and TSH are
low, this is consistent with a drug effect, secondary hypothyroidism, or the sick euthyroid
syndrome. Measurement of total T3 is not useful in evaluating a patient for hypothyroidism
because these levels are usually low normal
even in the face of significant hypothyroidism.
Antiepileptic drugs and salicylates typically
produce a low T4 level, yet these patients remain euthyroid with a normal TSH. Any acute
or chronic severe medical illness can cause the
sick euthyroid syndrome. These patients have
low total T4, low total T3, and normal TSH.
No clinical benefit has been shown from thyroxine replacement therapy in these patients.

Secondary hypothyroidism caused by pituitary or hypothalamic failure is usually suggested by other signs of panhypopituitarism.

D. Treatment.

L-thyroxine is the only appropriate replacement hormone for patients with hypothyroidism. The half-life is 7 days and it provides a steady level of the hormone. T3 (cytomel) has a very short half-life of 8 hours and is not useful as replacement therapy. T4/T3 combination medications are similarly not useful for replacement therapy. The replacement dose of L-thyroxine is variable from person to person but diminishes with age. Young patients generally need 0.125 to 0.15 mg/day whereas elderly patients generally need 0.075 to 0.1 mg/day. Serum T4 and TSH measurements are useful in follow-up dose adjustment.

E. Myxedema coma.

Myxedema coma is a medical emergency in which severe hypothyroid crisis is provoked by superimposed stress, often infection. Patients are generally elderly and present with hypotension, hypothermia, hypoventilation, respiratory failure, and coma. A vigorous therapeutic approach is necessary. Most patients should be intubated and placed on mechanical ventilation. Volume replacement guided by central venous pressure measurements is essential. Hypotension in the setting of myxedema is often insensitive to vasopressor drugs and should be treated with volume replacement instead. Patients with significant hypothermia should undergo passive rewarming. All patients should be given intravenous hydrocortisone (50–75 mg intravenously every 6 hours). Infection or other precipitating causes must be vigorously sought and treated. L-thyroxine is given intravenously with a loading bolus of 0.2–0.4 mg followed by 0.1 mg intravenously every day thereafter.

PITUITARY DISORDERS

I. Imaging.

Computed tomography (CT) with direct coronal views or magnetic resonance (MR) imaging are the techniques of choice for imaging the sella and pituitary gland.

II. Panhypopituitarism.

   A. Acute.

       1. Postpartum Sheehan's syndrome.

       2. Trauma.

       3. Meningitis.

       4. Rupture of an internal carotid aneurysm.

       5. Postoperative.

       6. Apoplexy (hemorrhage of a pituitary tumor).

   B. Chronic.

       1. Tuberculosis, fungal infections, syphilis.

       2. Radiation.

       3. Primary or metastatic tumors.

       4. Sarcoidosis or hemochromatosis.

       5. Hand-Schüller-Christian syndrome.

       6. Autoimmune hypophysitis.

   C. Signs and symptoms.

The signs and symptoms of panhypopituitarism are a composite of the various hormonal deficiencies. Patients often complain primarily of fatigue. Gonadal failure typically causes impotence and amenorrhea. Failure of lactation is a typical feature of postpartum hypopituitarism. However, in most patients with hypopituitarism, the symptoms are subtle and develop very insidiously, therefore, a high index of suspicion is necessary in identifying these patients.

   D. Diagnosis and laboratory evaluation.

       1. Thyroid gland:

The T4 measurement is usually low or low-normal. The total T3 measurement is usually normal. The TSH measurement is low or normal. Antithyroid antibodies are typically absent, and there is no response of TSH to TRH stimulation.

2. Adrenal gland:

The serum cortisol level is low or low-normal.
The ACTH level is usually low-normal. The initial screening test of choice for evaluating the
pituitary-adrenal axis is the rapid cortrosyn
stimulation test in which serum cortisol and aldosterone are measured at 0 and 60 minutes
after administration of an intravenous bolus of
0.25 mg cortrosyn. A stimulated serum cortisol
of greater than 20 is generally regarded as normal. Patients with primary or secondary adrenal
insufficiency will have a subnormal response of
serum cortisol to cortrosyn. However, a normal
stimulation of aldosterone is present in secondary adrenal insufficiency. The serum ACTH
level should be very elevated in primary adrenal insufficiency and low-normal in secondary
adrenal insufficiency and thus can also be quite
helpful. Additionally, the ability of the pituitary
gland to secrete ACTH can be tested with insu-
lin-induced hypoglycemia or metapyrone.

3. Gonadal function:

Hypopituitarism results in a low serum testosterone level, a low sperm count, and low LH
and FSH levels in men. In women, estradiol,
LH, and FSH levels are low. In both men and
women, there is no response of FSH and LH to
a rapid infusion of gonadatropin-releasing hormone (GNRH).

E. Treatment.

The treatment of pituitary failure involves replacement with thyroxine and cortisone as well as either
estrogen or testosterone. It is important to remember
that in patients with panhypopituitarism, cortisone
replacement must always precede thyroid hormone
replacement. Thyroid hormone replacement must
never be given to patients with a low T4 and a low
TSH level, as these patients may have unsuspected
panhypopituitarism and thyroid replacement therapy

can precipitate life-threatening adrenal insufficiency. Cortisone acetate 25 mg in the morning and 12.5 mg in the evening, and L-thyroxin 0.1 to 0.15 mg/day is standard replacement therapy. Patients with secondary adrenal insufficiency due to pituitary failure do not require mineralocorticoid replacement with Florinef.

III. Hypercortisolism: Cushing's syndrome.
 A. Etiology.
  1. Pituitary microadenoma (Cushing's disease) (70%).
  2. Adrenal adenoma or carcinoma (15%).
  3. Ectopic ACTH syndrome (15%).
 B. Signs and symptoms.
  1. Truncal obesity.
  2. Proximal muscle weakness and atrophy.
  3. Hypertension.
  4. Acne and hirsutism.
  5. Depression or psychosis.
  6. Plethora.
  7. Oligomenorrhea.
  8. Easy bruiseability.
  9. Osteopenia.
  10. Violatious striae.
  Routine laboratory abnormalities include hyperglycemia and hypokalemic alkalosis.
 C. Diagnosis.
  The overnight dexamethasone suppression test or the 24-hour urinary free cortisol test are reliable screening tests for hypercortisolism. One milligram of dexamethasone is given orally at midnight and at 8 A.M. the next morning, the serum cortisol is measured. Values greater than 5 are abnormal and suggest hypercortisolism. False-positive suppression tests occur in patients with depression, obesity, alcoholism, and in patients who are under severe stress. The 24-hour urinary free cortisol measurement is often normal in patients with obesity; however, depression and alcoholism are important

mimics of true hypercortisolism. Patients with hypercortisolism are evaluated next with the administration of 2 mg of dexamethasone every 6 hours for 48 hours and then measuring serum cortisol or a 24-hour urinary free cortisol. Alternatively, 8 mg of dexamethasone may be given as a single dose at midnight and the serum cortisol measurement obtained at 8 A.M. the next morning. Cortisol measurements that are suppressed greater than 50% of baseline are consistent with the diagnosis of a pituitary microadenoma. The autonomous adrenal secretion of cortisol generally shows no suppression with high dose dexamethasone. Patients with the ectopic ACTH syndrome also generally show less than 50% suppression with high dose dexamethasone. However, patients with ectopic ACTH secreted by a bronchial carcinoid tumor may suppress greater than 50% after high-dose dexamethasone, mimicking the response seen in pituitary microadenomas. ACTH levels are useful in differentiating autonomous adrenal tumors from ACTH-secreting tumors. In the former, ACTH levels are generally very low. In pituitary microadenomas, the ACTH levels are generally in the high-normal to somewhat elevated range. In patients with the ectopic ACTH syndrome, the ACTH levels may overlap those seen in pituitary microadenoma but are often substantially elevated. Once the diagnosis has been made biochemically, the next step is to localize the tumor with imaging techniques. In patients with pituitary microadenomas, CT scanning or MR imaging of the pituitary gland can be performed. However, 50% of patients who will subsequently be cured with transphenoidal surgery will have a normal-appearing pituitary gland with these imaging techniques. An adrenal tumor will generally be easily localized with abdominal CT scanning. However, caution must be exercised in interpreting such scans since approximately 5% of the normal population has a nonfunctioning benign adrenal adenoma easily depicted by CT. Thus, the hormonal diagnosis of adrenal autonomous hypercortisolism must be established before CT is performed so as not to be misled by the finding of an adrenal mass. Most tumors causing the ectopic ACTH syndrome can be localized within the chest with CT.

ADRENAL INSUFFICIENCY

The most common cause of adrenal insufficiency occurs in patients who have been chronically taking exogenous corticosteroids. It generally takes 6 to 12 months for the hypothalamic-pituitary-adrenal axis to recover from chronic exogenous steroid suppression. Stress during this time always has the potential to provoke adrenal insufficiency. The rapid cortrosyn stimulation test is useful for identifying inadequate adrenal reserve in such patients. Pending results, patients who are under stress must receive steroid coverage with hydrocortisone as described below.

   I. Primary adrenal insufficiency (Addison's disease).
        A. Signs and symptoms.
              1. Acute.
                    a. Hypotension.
                    b. Confusion.
                    c. Anorexia, nausea, and vomiting.
                    d. Abdominal pain.
                    e. Hyperthermia.
              2. Chronic.
                    a. Weakness.
                    b. Weight loss.
                    c. Anorexia.
                    d. Orthostasis.
                    e. Salt craving.
                    f. Abdominal pain.
                    g. Hyperpigmentation.
        B. Acute causes.
              1. Congenital adrenal hyperplasia in infants.
              2. Adrenal hemorrhage often secondary to anticoagulants.

3. Adrenal infarction, secondary to hypotension, often perioperative.
4. Adrenal infarction, secondary to overwhelming sepsis (Waterhouse-Friderichsen syndrome).

C. Chronic causes.

1. Autoimmune adrenal destruction accounts for 70% of all primary adrenal insufficiency. This is associated with hypoparathyroidism, Hashimoto's disease, type I diabetes, pernicious anemia, and hypogonadism.
2. Tuberculosis still accounts for 10% to 15% of cases of primary adrenal insufficiency.
3. Primary or metastatic malignancy.
4. Amyloidosis or hemochromatosis.
5. Surgical resection.
6. Drugs such as mitotane and aminoglutethamide.

D. Diagnosis.

The typical laboratory findings of primary adrenal insufficiency include: hyponatremia in 88% of patients, hyperkalemia in 65%, anemia, hypoglycemia, hypercalcemia, azotemia, eosinophilia, and lymphocytosis. Serum cortisol and aldosterone levels are extremely low and both show no response to the rapid 60-minute intravenous cortrosyn stimulation test.

F. Treatment.

If the patient is not critically ill, then a 60-minute cortrosyn stimulation test should be performed prior to initiation of intravenous cortisone therapy. A cortisol level greater than 20 after administration of cortrosyn is considered normal. Hydrocortisone (100 mg intravenously every 6 hours or a continuous infusion at 20 mg/hr) is begun. Normal saline must be infused to correct the typical volume deficit. Acute adrenal insufficiency is most typically provoked by superimposed stress, such as infection, which must be actively sought and treated. Once the patient has become stable, the dose of hydrocortisone can be tapered to maintenance oral therapy, which is cortisone acetate 25 mg A.M., 12.5 mg in the P.M., or hydrocortisone 20 mg in the A.M., 10 mg in P.M., or prednisone 5 mg in the A.M., 2.5 mg in the P.M., or dexamethasone 1 mg A.M.. Intravenous hydrocortisone has adequate mineralocorticoid activity at doses of 200–400 mg/day; however, maintenance glucocorticoids possess very little mineralocorticoid activity. Thus, the oral mineralocorticoid florinef (0.05 mg to 0.2 mg/day) must also be included. Patients with adrenal insufficiency undergoing surgery should receive 100 mg of hydrocortisone intravenously every 6 hours beginning 6 hours prior to surgery. After 24 to 36 hours, the dose may taper to maintenance over the next 3 to 4 days as long as a stressful postoperative complication does not intervene.

ENDOCRINE CAUSES OF HYPERTENSION

The endocrine causes of hypertension are rare. Renal vascular disease causes 2% of hypertension, pheochromocytoma causes 0.1% of hypertension, and primary hyperaldosteronism causes 0.5% of hypertension. These surgically curable causes of hypertension should be sought in patients in whom hypertension develops at a young age, in whom hypertension is refractory to significant pharmacologic therapy, and those with a history of paroxsyms or who have significant hypokalemia.

I. Renal vascular disease.
   A. Clinical clues.
      1. Extensive atherosclerotic disease in older patients.
      2. A midabdominal bruit.
      3. Hypokalemia occurs in approximately 20% of patients.
   B. Etiology.
      1. Atherosclerotic stenosis of one or both renal arteries in older patients.
      2. Fibromuscular dysplasia of one renal artery in younger patients.

C. Diagnostic approach.

The captopril stimulation test as devised by Laragh et al. is the recommended first screening test for renal artery stenosis. To perform the test, all antihypertensive drugs and diuretics should be stopped for at least a week. *This should only be done with extreme caution* since the patient may develop significant hypertension if antihypertensive therapy is discontinued. The test is not accurate if the serum creatinine level is greater than 2. Patients should be on a high salt diet for a few days prior to the test and a 24-hour urine sodium level must be greater than 60 mEq prior to proceeding with the test. Patients who are volume depleted with a low urine sodium will have a false-positive test result. This test has greater than 95% diagnostic accuracy as long as the patient has a normal BUN and creatinine, and as long as the patient is euvolemic. The next step is to confirm the diagnosis and localize the lesion with renal arteriography.

D. Treatment.

Percutaneous transluminal balloon angioplasty has now become the first treatment of choice for most patients with renal artery stenosis. Patients in whom percutaneous angioplasty is unsuccessful will require surgical revascularization.

II. Pheochromocytoma.

A. Signs and symptoms.

Approximately 50% of patients with pheochromocytoma will give a history of paroxsymal attacks. Typical symptoms of such a paroxymal attack include severe headache, tachycardia, tremor, sweating, and anxiety. Paroxsyms may be provoked by surgery (especially induction of general anesthesia), labor and delivery, intravenous contrast infusion, or sexual intercourse. The differential diagnosis of such paroxsyms includes: superventricular or ventricular tachyarrhythmias, migraines, thyrotoxicosis, panic attacks, angina, and hypoglycemia. The symptoms of a paroxsym associated with the carcinoid syndrome, flushing, wheezing, and diarrhea do not commonly overlap with those of pheochromocytoma. The remaining 50% of patients with pheochromocytoma have sustained severe hypertension. It is also common for patients with pheochromocytoma to have orthostatic hypotension. Indeed, the triad of hypertension, hypotension, and tachycardia in the same individual must always suggest pheochromocytoma.

B. Diagnostic approach.

Twenty four-hour urine collections may be performed. Vanillomandelic acid (VMA) measurement has a diagnostic sensitivity of approximately 40% to 50%. Metanephrine measurement has a diagnostic sensitivity of approximately 80%. Urinary norepinephrine and epinephrine measurements have a diagnostic sensitivity around 80%. Twenty four-hour urine specimens may be inaccurate because of problems with incomplete urine collection. The vast majority of patients with pheochromocytoma have sustained hypercatecholaminemia whether their hypertension is sustained or paroxsymal. For these reasons, plasma norepinephrine and epinephrine measurements are often used. A single plasma measurement has a diagnostic sensitivity between 90% and 95%. The patient must be resting quietly and an indwelling intravenous catheter must be in place for at least 30 minutes prior to obtaining the sample for plasma catecholamines. The blood is drawn into a prechilled heparinized tube and rapidly transported to the laboratory on ice where it should be promptly separated and frozen. Occasionally, patients with pheochromocytoma will have plasma catecholamine levels that overlap with essential hypertension in the 800–1,500 pg/mL range. These results may be delineated with the use of clonidine. Clonidine will suppress the production of plasma catecholamines in essential hypertension whereas catecholamine production by a pheochromocytoma will not be affected. A sample is obtained for plasma catecholamine measurement before and 3 hours after the ingestion of 0.3 mg of clonidine. Once the diagnosis of pheochromocytoma is made on the basis of significant catecholamine elevation, an abdominal CT scan or MR image will localize most tumors. Hypertensive crisis may be provoked in patients with unsuspected pheochromocytoma with general anesthesia, or at labor and delivery. In this event, the blood pressure may be safely controlled with an intravenous infusion of nitroprusside. Intravenous boluses of phentolamine may also be useful. β-blocking drugs (propranolol, labetolol) create a situation of unopposed α stimulation, which may exacerbate the hypertension of pheochromocytoma and thus are contraindicated in patients with pheochromocytoma who have not already received established α blockade. Phenoxybenzamine is the oral drug of choice for control of hypertension and preparation of patients with pheochromocytoma for surgery. The drug has a half-life of 24 hours. Generally, patients are begun on 10 mg orally every 12 hours and the dose is increased every 48 hours up to a range of 40–80 mg with careful monitoring of the blood pressure response. Since patients with pheochromocytoma usually have volume contraction, judicious intravenous volume expansion with crystalloid solutions and packed RBCs is an important part of preoperation preparation. Careful attention must be given to avoiding congestive heart failure in elderly patients. Patients with arrhythmias or residual tachycardia (greater than 100 beats per minute) after α blockade is established may benefit from propanolol, 10–20 mg orally every 6 hours.

III. Primary hyperaldosteronism.
    A. Clinical clues.

        Approximately 70% to 80% of patients with primary hyperaldosteronism have significant hypokalemia with potassium values less than 3.0. Other diseases in which hypokalemia and hypertension are associated include renal artery stenosis and Cushing's syndrome.

B. Diagnostic approach.

There are two basic criteria that must be met to diagnose hyperaldosteronism: plasma renin must be unstimulatable, and serum aldosterone must be nonsuppressable. All antihypertensive drugs and diuretics must be stopped if possible for at least a week prior to testing. Renin may be stimulated either by giving furosemide 40 mg intravenously and maintaining an upright posture for 2 hours or by giving 50 mg of Captopril. Plasma renin is measured 2 hours after either one of these maneuvers. Patients with primary hyperaldosteronism will generally have plasma renin values less than 1 after either one of these maneuvers. Serum aldosterone is suppressed by the physiologic maneuver of volume expansion. Two liters of 0.9% NaCl is infused over 4 hours. Serum aldosterone is normally suppressed to less than 8 ng/mL by this maneuver. A value significantly greater than this when accompanied by a suppressed plasma renin value is diagnostic of primary hyperaldosteronism. Once the diagnosis is established, abdominal CT will facilitate identification of patients who have a single adrenal adenoma, which can then be surgically resected. Approximately 40% of patients with primary hyperaldosteronism have bilateral adrenal hyperplasia. These patients and occasional patients with unilateral adenoma who are not surgical candidates will need to be treated medically. In most patients, hypertension can be controlled with either spironolactone 25–100 mg orally every 6 hours or amiloride 10–40 mg per day. Many patients also need a calcium-channel blocker such as nifedipine 10–30 mg orally every 6 hours.

DISORDERS OF CALCIUM REGULATION

I. Hypercalcemia.

A. Signs and symptoms.

1. Weakness.
2. Anorexia.
3. Nausea, vomiting.
4. Mental status changes.
5. Coma.
6. Polyuria.
7. Constipation.
8. Kidney stones.
9. Osteoporosis.
10. Often is asymptomatic.

B. Etiology.
   1. Primary hyperparathyroidism accounts for approximately 70% of all hypercalcemia. It is often discovered on routine blood testing of asymptomatic patients.
   2. Many different malignancies may be associated with hypercalcemia. Many solid tumors, especially squamous cell tumors, produce a peptide that has similar biologic activity to that of parathyroid hormone. However, this hormone is immunologically different from parathyroid hormone and thus is not measured in parathyroid hormone assays. Multiple myeloma produces hypercalcemia by the local production of osteoclast-activating factors. Other malignancies, such as breast cancer, likely produce hypercalcemia by direct and diffuse bone invasion and destruction. In all forms of hypercalcemia associated with malignancy, intact parathyroid hormone levels are normal or suppressed.
   3. Thiazides, lithium, tamoxifen, and aluminum can cause hypercalcemia.
   4. Hyperthyroidism and adrenal insufficiency have been associated with hypercalcemia.
   5. Familial hypocalciuric hypercalcemia is an autosomal dominant defect in renal calcium excretion and is a benign entity requiring no treatment. Parathyroid hormone levels may be normal or slightly elevated. This entity can be diagnosed in patients with mild hypercalcemia

by finding a very low 24-hour urine calcium measurement. All other forms of hypercalcemia except perhaps patients on thiazide diuretics will have an elevated 24-hour urine calcium measurement.

6. Vitamin D excess. There are two basic mechanisms by which patients may have vitamin D toxicity and hypercalcemia. Patients may take excessive doses of a pharmacologic vitamin D preparation. Alternatively, patients may have one of a variety of granulomatous diseases, including sarcoidosis, tuberculosis, histoplasmosis, as well as lymphoma. In these diseases, the macrophages within the granulomas possess the 1-α-hydroxylase enzyme for the conversion of 25-hydroxy vitamin D to the active 1, 25-dihydroxy vitamin D. The hypercalcemia of vitamin D excess is sensitive to inhibition by low doses of glucocorticoids. Patients are given 20–30 mg of prednisone orally per day for 5 days. This treatment will normalize the serum calcium levels in patients who have underlying vitamin D excess.

C. Diagnostic evaluation.

Patients with an underlying malignancy that is known to be associated with hypercalcemia do not present a diagnostic difficulty. Vitamin D preparations or thiazide diuretics should be discontinued. Hyperthyroidism and adrenal insufficiency must be sought if suggested by clinical clues. In the remainder of patients with hypercalcemia, the next step is to measure levels of intact parathyroid hormone. An assay of the intact hormone is preferable to an assay of hormone fragments. In general, the degree of hypercalcemia correlates well with the degree of elevation of intact parathyroid hormone levels. Patients with hypercalcemia who have no evidence of malignancy, no history of thiazide or vitamin D use, and normal parathyroid hormone measurements should undergo a 24-hour urine calcium measurement, assessment of thyroid and adrenal function, and a steroid suppression test as described above.

D. Treatment.

Most patients with mild hypercalcemia are asymtomatic and do not require emergent treatment. However, as calcium levels rise, the likelihood of significant symptoms also rises. Calcium levels in excess of 18 mg/dL usually cause mental status changes, dehydration, and renal insufficiency, and constitute a medical emergency known as hypercalcemic crisis. Therapy depends on the severity of hypercalcemia and the degree to which the patient is symptomatic. Most patients with significant hypercalcemia are dehydrated and volume expansion with 0.9% NaCl is essential. They may be given 200–500 mL/hr of 0.9% NaCl. Additionally, furosemide can further enhance caliuresis. Once initial rehydration is complete, patients may be given 40–80 mg of furosemide intravenously every 6 hours. Consequently, a brisk diuresis will ensue and careful attention must be paid to sodium and potassium levels as well as to fluid balance. Patients with hypercalcemic crisis should also be immediately given intravenous mithramycin at a dose of 25 mg/kg daily for 3 days. Its toxicity includes bone marrow suppression and nephrotoxicity. Patients with hypercalcemic crisis who do not have a prompt response to mithramycin or patients who have developed acute renal insufficiency secondary to hypercalcemia should undergo dialysis. The drug ediotronate is effective in controlling the hypercalcemia of malignancy. It is given intravenously at a dose of 7.5 mg/kg daily for 3 days. As previously discussed, low dose glucocorticoids are the treatment of choice for hypercalcemia secondary to vitamin D excess. Some patients with hypercalcemia secondary to breast cancer or multiple myeloma may also respond to high-dose steroids (60–100 mg/day of prednisone or its equivalent). Occasionally, calcitonin 100–200 units intramuscularly or subcutaneously every 12 hours is a useful adjunct to steroids in these patients. In general, the long-term outcome of patients with hypercalcemia is linked to the success with which their underlying disease can be treated. Treatment of mild asymptomatic hyperparathyroidism is controversial. Many post menopausal women can be effectively treated with estrogen therapy. Premarin (0.625–1.25 mg/day) often will normalize the serum calcium level. Oral phosphate therapy (neutrophoas two tablets orally three times a day) may also be a useful adjunct, especially in patients with kidney stones. Most patients with hyperparathyroidism and sustained serum calcium levels greater than 11.5 should be referred for parathyroid surgery.

II. Hypocalcemia disorders.
  A. Signs and symptoms.
     The clinical manifestations of hypocalcemia include muscle cramps, tetany, psychosis, laryngospasm, seizures, and death. Carpopedal spasm after inflation of a blood pressure cuff above systolic pressure for 3 minutes (Trousseau's sign) may predict impending hypocalcemic crisis. Facial nerve irritability (Chvostek's sign) may also be present but is less specific. Intractable congestive heart failure and/or hypotension are being increasingly recognized as important manifestations of severe hypocalcemia.
  B. Etiology.
     1. Hypoparathyroidism after thyroid or parathyroid surgery: hypocalcemia followed by hyperphosphatemia usually develops within 48 hours in affected patients.
     2. "Hungry bones" syndrome occurs in patients with longstanding hyperthyroidism or hyperparathyroidism after surgical resection of the thyroid or parathyroid glands. These patients with postoperative hypocalcemia do not develop hyperphosphatemia, which distinguishes them from those with hypoparathyroidism.

    3. Hypomagnesemia. This may commonly be caused by thiazides, cisplatinum, cyclosporine, chronic alcoholism, or poor nutrition. Serum magnesium is required both for the release and action of parathyroid hormone and thus, hypocalcemia may ensue.

    4. Malabsorption can cause vitamin D deficiency, hypocalcemia, and hypophosphatemia.

    5. Sepsis. Recent data indicate that as many as 50% of patients with overwhelming gram-positive or gram-negative sepsis may develop significant hypocalcemia.

    6. Acute pancreatitis.

    7. Idiopathic hypoparathyroidism. This is an autoimmune disease associated with autoimmune hypothyroidism and adrenal insufficiency. Serum phosphate levels are elevated.

    8. Pseudohypoparathyroidism is an inherited syndrome in which patients are severely resistant to parathyroid hormone. They have a typical somatic appearance including short stature, obesity, and shortened fourth metacarpals and metatarsals. Approximately 50% of the patients also have primary hypothyroidism.

C. Diagnosis.

All patients with suspected hypocalcemia should be evaluated with measurement of free ionized calcium, serum phosphorous, and serum magnesium. Patients with pseudohypoparathyroidism will have very elevated intact parathyroid hormone measurements, and values in most other patients with hypocalcemia will be normal or low. All patients with hypoparathyroidism should be hyperphosphatemic. Hungry bones syndrome, pancreatitis, and sepsis all cause combined hypocalcemia and hypophosphatemia, but usually do not present a diagnostic dilemma. Hypocalcemia and hypophosphatemia in most other patients is caused by malabsorption and vitamin D deficiency.

D. Treatment.

All patients with acute severe hypocalcemia with or without symptoms should be treated with intravenous calcium replacement. Be extremely cautious in patients with pancreatitic, toxic shock syndrome, and rhabdomyolysis since they may have rebound hypercalcemia with resolution of these disorders. Ten milliliters of 10% calcium chloride is the preferred calcium salt and should be given as a 20 to 30 minute intravenous infusion every 1 to 2 hours in symptomatic patients and every 6 to 12 hours in asymptomatic patients with careful monitoring of serum calcium levels. Thirty milliliters of 10% calcium gluconate will deliver an equivalent dose of elemental calcium. Chronic asymptomatic hypocalcemia does not generally constitute a medical emergency and most patients can be treated with oral calcium replacement. Calcium carbonate 500–1,000 mg orally every 8 hours or calcium citrate 3,000 mg orally every 8 hours are usually effective doses. All patients with hypoparathyroidism will also require vitamin D therapy for normalization of serum calcium levels. Vitamin D2 (ergocalciferol) is cheap, effective, chronic therapy, and the usual dose is 50,000 units per day. Since it has a half-life of 4 weeks, it may take 4 to 8 weeks before its effects are seen. The active metabolite of vitamin D, 1, 25-dihydroxy-vitamin D, has a very short half-life of 12 to 24 hours and is often used to bridge the gap in initiating chronic vitamin D therapy. The usual dose is 0.5–1.5 mg/day. Magnesium deficiency should be corrected with an intravenous infusion over 30 minutes of 2 g of magnesium sulfate every 12 hours until serum magnesium levels are normalized. Patients with hypocalcemia and hypomagnesemia will not respond to calcium replacement until the magnesium deficiency is corrected.

BIBLIOGRAPHY

Felig P, et al: *Endocrinology and Metabolism*, ed 2. New York, McGraw-Hill Book Co, 1987.

Marble A, et al: *Joslin's Diabetes Mellitus*, ed 12. Philadelphia, Lea & Febiger, 1985.

Lavin N: *Manual of Endocrinology and Metabolism*. St Louis, Little Brown, 1986.

Bardin CW: *Current Therapy in Endocrinology*. Toronto, Canada, BC Decker, 1988.

Thyroid Disorders

Cooper DS: Antithyroid drugs. *N Engl J Med* 1984; 311:1353–1362.

Robuschi G, et al: Hypothyroidism in the elderly. *Endocr Rev* 1987; 8:142–153.

Hoffenberg R: Thyroid emergencies. *Clin Endocrinol Metab* 1980; 9:503–512.

Diabetes Mellitus and Hypoglycemia

Eisenbarth G: Type I diabetes mellitus: A chronic autoimmune disease. *N Engl J Med* 1986; 314:1360–1368.

Foster DW, McGarry JD: The metabolic derangements and treatment of diabetic ketoacidosis. *N Engl J Med* 1983; 309:159–169.

Gerich JE: Sulfonylureas in the treatment of diabetes mellitus: 1985. *Mayo Clin Proc* 1985; 60:439–443.

Arieff AI, Carroll HJ: Nonketotic hyperosmolar coma with hyperglycemia: Clinical features, pathophysiology, renal function, acid-base balance, plasma-cerebrospinal fluid equilibria and the effects of therapy in 37 cases. *Medicine* 1972; 51:73–94.

Raskin P, Rosenstock J: Blood glucose control and diabetic complications. *Ann Intern Med* 1986; 105:254–263.

Nelson RL: Hypoglycemia: Fact or fiction? *Mayo Clin Proc* 1985; 60:844–850.

Pituitary and Adrenal Disorders

Abboud CF: Laboratory diagnosis of hypopituitarism. *Mayo Clin Proc* 1986; 61:35–48.

Carpenter PC: Cushing's syndrome: Update of diagnosis and management. *Mayo Clin Proc* 1986; 61:49–58.

May ME, Carey RM: Rapid adrenocorticotropic hormone test in practice: Retrospective review. *Am J Med* 1985; 79:679–684.

Burke CW: Adrenocortical insufficiency. *Clin Endocrinol Metab* 1985; 14:947–975.

Endocrine Causes of Hypertension

Vaughan ED: Renovascular hypertension. *Kidney Int* 1985; 27:811–827.

Bravo EL, Gifford RW: Pheochromocytoma: Diagnosis, localization and management. *N Engl J Med* 1984; 311:1297–1304.

Streeten DH, Tomycz N, Anderson GH: Reliability of screening methods for the diagnosis of primary aldosteronism. *Am J Med* 1979; 67:403–413.

Calcium Disorders

Klee GG, Kao PC, Heath H: Hypercalcemia. *Endocrinol Metab Clin N Am* 1988; 17:573–599.

Stewart AF: Therapy of malignancy-associated hypercalcemia: 1983. *Am J Med* 1983; 74:475–480.

Zaloga GP, Chernow B: Hypocalcemia in critical illness. *JAMA* 1986; 256:1924–1929.

Neurology

11

Aaron Hamb, M.D.
Mark Dietz, M.D.
Susan Nadis, M.D.
Nina Paleologos, M.D.
Michael Rezak, M.D.

COMA

I. Definition.

Coma is a state of unarousable psychologic unresponsiveness in which the subject lies with eyes closed. Subjects in coma show no psychologically understandable response to external stimulus or inner need. To produce a coma, lesions must involve both cerebral hemispheres, the ascending reticular activating system, or both.

II. History.

It is important to determine if the patient's decreased level of consciousness has occurred acutely or gradually over time. A history of head trauma, which may have lead to acute epidural bleeding, or slow subdural bleeding is of prognostic and therapeutic importance. A patient with a history of diabetes mellitus may have diabetic ketoacidosis or hyperosmolar nonketotic coma. The patient should be examined for needle-track marks since drug overdose is a more common cause of coma in the young. A history of renal disease or hepatic failure may help to define a metabolic cause of decreased consciousness. Obviously, the history will need to be obtained from previous medical records and most importantly from family or significant others.

III. Physical examination.

    A. Coma examination.

        1. Vital signs and respiratory pattern (Fig 11–1).

        2. Observe and examine pupils (Fig 11–2).

        3. Corneal reflex.

        4. Observe for spontaneous eye movements.

        5. Oculocephalic reflex (Doll's eyes) and oculo-vestibular reflex (Fig 11–3).

        6. Localization of painful stimuli.

        7. Observe spontaneous posturing and posturing after stimulation (Fig 11–4).

One must determine whether or not the patient's decreased level of consciousness is associated with focal or localized findings (Table 11–1). This suggests a focal structural abnormality as opposed to a more generalized metabolic defect. This is not an absolute rule, and metabolic defects such as hypoglycemia have been known to masquerade as focal seizures.

IV. Reversible causes of coma.

Whenever you are presented with a patient in a coma, all reversible causes must be ruled out. These include electrolyte abnormalities, hypoglycemia, Wernicke's encephalopathy, narcotic drug overdose, infection (especially in a febrile patient with nuchal rigidity), and trauma. The following should serve as a guide to diagnostic screening and empiric therapy of the patient at initial presentation. This is not a substitute for a thorough history and physical examination.

    A. Draw stat electrolyte and glucose levels, drug and toxin screens, and complete blood cell (CBC) count.

    B. Administer universal antidotes.

        1. One ampule D50 (or 1 mg/kg D50) intravenously.

        2. Thiamine 100 mg intravenously.

        3. Naloxone 0.8 mg intravenously: slow push. Patients have gone into acute withdrawal with this therapy.

        4. Oxygen.

        5. Antidotes should be administered for specific toxins when identified.

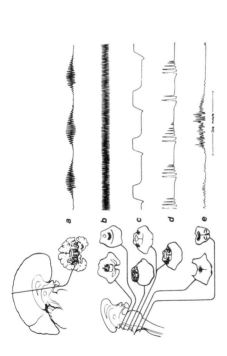

FIG 11–1
Abnormal respiratory patterns associated with pathologic lesions (shaded areas) at various levels of the brain. Tracings by chest-abdomen pneumograph, inspiration reads up. **a**, Cheyne-Stokes respiration. **b**, central neurogenic hyperventilation. **c**, apneusis. **d**, cluster breathing. **e**, ataxic breathing. (From Plum F, Posner JB: *The Diagnosis of Stupor and Coma*, ed 3. Philadelphia, FA Davis Co, 1982. Used by permission.)

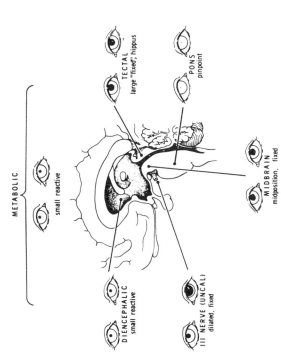

FIG 11–2
Pupils in comatose patients. (From Plum F, Posner JB: *The Diagnosis of Stupor and Coma*, ed 3. Philadelphia, FA Davis Co, 1982. Used by permission.)

6. A lumbar puncture should be performed if meningitis is suspected and there are no focal neurological findings. If focal abnormalities are present, computed tomography (CT) should be performed to assess the likelihood of cerebral herniation with a lumbar puncture.

C. Obtain a stat CT scan of the brain if trauma or focal neurologic findings are found.

V. Differential diagnosis.

A. Cerebrovascular accident.
   1. Intracerebral hemorrhage.
   2. Aneurysmal rupture with subarachnoid hemorrhage.
   3. Large hemispheral infarction.
   4. Brain stem infarction (coma vs. locked in syndrome) vide infra.
   5. Multiple bilateral infarcts (emboli).

B. Head trauma.
   1. Increased intracranial pressure.
   2. Brain stem trauma.

C. Metabolic abnormalities.
   1. Hyper- or hyponatremia.
   2. Hyperglycemic hyperosmolar nonketotic coma.
   3. Uremic encephalopathy.
   4. Hepatic encephalopathy.
   5. Anoxia/hypoxia.
   6. Myxedema coma (hypothyroidism).
   7. Wernicke's encephalopathy.

D. Postoperative complications.
   Pseudocholinesterase deficiency results in a marked sensitivity to suxamethonium given as a muscle relaxant during anesthesia.

E. Intraoperative complications.
   1. Hypotension may lead to significant cerebral ischemia.
   2. Arrhythmias.
   3. Myocardial infarction.

VI. Conditions resembling coma.

A. Locked-in syndrome: a clinical state in which there

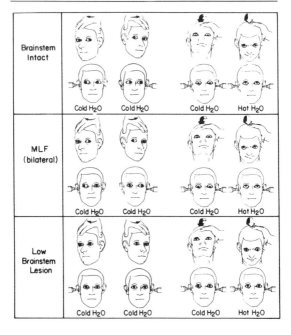

FIG 11–3

Ocular reflexes in unconscious patients. The upper section illustrates the oculocephalic (above) and oculovestibular (below) reflexes in an unconscious patient whose brain stem ocular pathways are intact. Horizontal eye movements are illustrated on the left and vertical eye movements on the right: lateral conjugated eye movements (upper left) to head turning are full and opposite in direction to the movement of the face. A stronger stimulus to lateral deviation is achieved by douching cold water against the tympanic membrane(s). There is tonic conjugate deviation of both eyes toward the stimulus; the eyes remain tonically deviated for 1 or more minutes before slowly returning to the midline. Because the patient is unconscious, there is no nystagmus. Extension of the neck in a patient with an intact brain stem produces deviation of the eyes upward. Bilateral cold water against the tympanic membrane likewise produces conjugate downward deviation of the eyes, whereas hot water (no warmer than 44°C) causes conjugate upward deviation of the eyes. In the middle portion of the drawing, the effects of bilateral medial longitudinal fasciculus lesion on oculocephalic and oculovestibular reflexes are shown. The left portion of the drawing illustrates that oculocephalic and oculovestibular stimulation deviates the appropriate eye laterally and brings the eye, which would normally deviate medially, only to the midline, since the medial longitudinal fasciculus, with its connections between the abducens and oculomotor nuclei, is interrupted. Vertical eye movements often remain intact. The lower portion of the drawing illustrates the effects of a low brain stem lesion. On the left, neither oculovestibular nor oculocephalic movements cause lateral deviation of the eyes because the pathways are interrupted between the vestibular nucleus and the abducens area. Likewise, in the right portion of the drawing, neither oculovestibular nor oculocephalic stimulation causes vertical deviation of the eyes. On rare occasions, particularly with low lateral brain stem lesions, oculocephalic responses may be intact even when oculovestibular reflexes are abolished. (From Plum F, Posner JB: *The Diagnosis of Stupor and Coma*, ed 3. Philadelphia, FA Davis Co, 1982. Used by permission.)

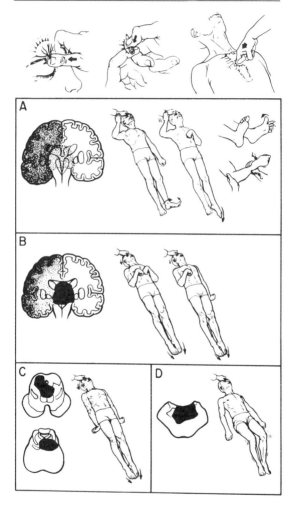

FIG 11–4

Motor responses to noxious stimulation in patients with acute cerebral dysfunction. Noxious stimuli can be delivered with minimal trauma to the supraorbital ridge, the nail bed, or the sternum as illustrated at the top. Levels of associated brain dysfunction are roughly indicated at the left. (From Plum F, Posner JB: *The Diagnosis of Stupor and Coma*, ed 3. Philadelphia, FA Davis Co, 1982. Used by permission.)

TABLE 11-1.
Localizing Signs in Coma

Site	Breathing	Pupils	Posture*
Hemispheres	Posthyperventilation apnea	Not helpful	Decorticate
Diencephalon	Cheyne-Stokes respiration (also with deep hemispheral lesions)	Horner's miosis	
Midbrain	Central neurogenic hyperventilation†	Midposition and fixed	Decerebrate
Pons	Apneustic	Pinpoint	Decerebrate
Medulla	Ataxic	Pinpoint	No posturing

†Rare.
*Similar signs may be seen at several levels.

      is little or no disturbance of awareness, but there is
an inability to respond.

  B. Akinetic mutism: a patient appears to be awake but
is unresponsive.

  C. Catatonia: condition in which the patient is motion-
less, completely without volition and without reaction to sensory stimuli.

VII. Brain death.

Legally this is a very complicated issue and definitions
are based on state laws. It is important to be familiar
with the laws in your state. Clinically this condition is
defined as the absence of both cerebral and brain stem
function. If any spontaneous functions exist, the patient
is not brain dead. Figure 11–5 is an example of the
Brain Death and Cadaver Organ Transplantation Criteria
for the New York Hospital.

VIII. Seizures.

  A. Definition.

A convulsive disorder that is the result of an acute,
excessive disorderly discharge of neurons from
either areas of grossly normal or structurally dis-
eased cortex. This results in spontaneous motor abnormalities which if generalized cause loss of
consciousness. A general discussion of the types of
seizures and their treatments is beyond the scope of
this book. Discussed here is the approach to a patient that is having a seizure. First determine if the
airway is compromised. This is most often the result
of the tongue resting in the posterior pharynx. The
head should be gently turned to the side to prevent
aspiration. If available, review the patient's history
for prior seizure activity and medication. If no history is available, the differential diagnosis is broad-
ened and should include electrolyte disturbances,
structural abnormalities, infarct, meningitis, hypoglycemia, and trauma as well as a primary seizure
disorder.

  B. History.

    1. Description of seizure: note that an aura is part

BRAIN DEATH

Brain death shall mean the irreversible loss of vital brain functions.

A person may be pronounced dead if it is determined by an attending physician, and confirmed in consultation by an attending neurologist, neurosurgeon, or anesthesiologist, that the individual has suffered Brain Death. When the person thought to be brain dead is under ten years of age, one of the two attending physicians must be a pediatric neurologist.*

Determination of Brain Death shall be made in accordance with the mandatory criteria listed below. All observations, tests, and findings shall be recorded in the patient's chart. Supplementary criteria may be used at the physician's discretion.

The consultant may either work with the primary attending physician in making the diagnosis of Brain Death or perform an independent confirmation which shall include review of the data and conclusions obtained by the primary attending physician and readministration of the testing required in section 2 below to determine no vital brain function. Only a single 12-hour period of no brain function, as provided below, need have elapsed in connection with the diagnosis of Brain Death by the primary attending and the consulting physicians.

The 12-hour period may be shortened to as little as 6 hours in cases of established irreversible structural damage provided that the mandatory clinical criteria are confirmed by one or more of the supplementary criteria.

I. MANDATORY CRITERIA
  A. Coma of Established Cause

FIG 11–5

Brain death and cadaver organ transplantation criteria for the New York Hospital. (From Plum F, Posner JB: *The Diagnosis of Stupor and Coma,* ed 3: Philadelphia, FA Davis Co, 1982. Used by permission.)

    1. No potentially anesthetizing amounts of either toxins or therapeutic drugs can be present; hypothermia below 30°C or other physiologic abnormalities must be corrected to the extent medically possible.

    2. Irreversible structural disease or a known and irreversible endogenous metabolic cause due to organ failure must be present.

B. A 12-Hour Period of No Brain Function Must Have Elapsed:

    1. No Cerebral Function
    No behavioral or reflex response involving structures above the cervical spinal cord can be elicited by noxious stimuli delivered anywhere in the body.

    2. No Brainstem Reflexes
      a. The pupils must be fixed to light.
      b. No corneal reflexes can be present.
      c. There must be no response to icewater calorics (50 ml. in each ear).
      d. No spontaneous respirations must occur during apneic oxygenation for a period of 10 minutes.
      e. The circulation may be intact.
      f. Purely spinal cord reflexes may be retained.

II. SUPPLEMENTARY CRITERIA

A. An EEG for 30 minutes at maximal gain reflects absence of cerebral electrical activity.

B. Brainstem auditory or short latency somatic evoked responses reflect absence of function in vital brainstem structures.

C. No cerebral circulation present on angiographic examination.

---

*This paragraph emphasizes the importance of experienced consultation in critical medical decisions that involved social-humanistic as well as scientific considerations. The choice of consultants reflects local experience but the principle lends dignity to the act of diagnosis and minimizes the risk of future doubts by all concerned.

of the seizure and often an indication of the focus of initial discharge.
    a. Sequence of spread.
    b. Lateralizing signs during and after seizure.
    c. Presence/absence of smells, tastes, hallucinations, automatisms.
  2. Family history.
  3. Past medical history.
    a. Signs/symptoms of infection.
    b. Metabolic disorders.
    c. Past trauma.
    d. Previous cerebrovascular accident.
  4. Birth history.
  5. Drug and/or alcohol abuse.
C. General physical examination.
  1. Blood pressure, pulse, temperature.
  2. Signs of peripheral emboli.
  3. Skin examination.
  4. Signs of drug withdrawal.
D. Neurologic examinations.
  May show some lateralization.
E. Etiology.
  1. Congenital (primary congenital, birth trauma).
  2. Infectious (meningitis, encephalitis, brain abscess).
  3. Trauma (acute head injury, post-traumatic, subdural or epidural hematoma).
  4. Metabolic (sodium, calcium, water intoxication, dehydration, uremia, hepatic encephalopathy, hyper- or hypoglycemia, anoxia).
  5. Toxic (carbon monoxide, lead, mercury, alcohol, barbiturate, theophylline, tricyclic antidepressants, lidocaine).
  6. Cerebrovascular (subarachnoid hemorrhage, postinfarct, embolus, hypertensive encephalopathy, arteriovenous malformation, vasculitis).
  7. Neoplasm (primary in brain, metastatic).
  8. Idiopathic.
F. Laboratory evaluation.
  1. Blood work.

   a. CBC, sedimentation rate.
   b. Electrolyte levels, specifically sodium, calcium, magnesium.
   c. Toxin screen, specific drug/alcohol levels.
   d. Anticonvulsant levels.
   e. Glucose level.
   f. Arterial blood gas.
   g. Blood urea nitrogen, creatinine.
   h. Liver function tests.
2. Radiologic evaluation.
   CT scan: without infusion, and then if no hemorrhage is present, with infusion.
3. Spinal tap: cell count, glucose, protein, gram stain, cultures, syphillis serology, cytology if carcinoma suspected.
4. Other.
   a. Electrocardiogram.
   b. Electroencephalogram: need not be obtained immediately unless subclinical status epilepticus is suspected.

G. Status epilepticus.
   Generalized status epilepticus is defined as prolonged (30 minutes or longer) convulsions, or convulsions that are so frequent that each attack begins before the postictal period of the preceding one ends. General management:
   1. Maintain adequate airway and oxygenation.
   2. Obtain blood samples for diagnostic studies and anticonvulsant levels.
   3. Administer thiamine 100 mg intravenously in an unknown patient and in patients with suspected alcohol abuse and/or nutritional deficits.
   4. Administer glucose 25–50 g (in adults) via rapid intravenous infusion.
   5. Treatment should include restoration of therapeutic levels of anticonvulsant drugs if the patient has been noncompliant. For immediate control, Lorazepam 1 mg intravenously may be administered every 2 to 3 minutes until the sei-

zure stops. If this proves ineffective after a few doses, phenytoin (15–18 mg/kg) slow IV push (50 mg/min) should be administered. If the seizure continues to persist, phenobarbitol 120–240 mg, given slow IV push, is administered. This is repeated at 30-minute intervals with a total dosage of 5–10 mg/kg. If no response, 8–10 ml of paraldehyde mixed with an equal volume of vegetable oil (per rectum) is recommended. A rubber catheter for the retention enema should be used since paraldehyde reacts with plastics. If seizures persist the patient should receive general anesthesia.

BIBLIOGRAPHY

Adams RD, Victor M: *Principles of Neurology*, ed 2. New York, McGraw-Hill Book Co, 1981.
Plum F, Posner JB: *The Diagnosis of Stupor and Coma*, ed 3. Philadelphia, FA Davis Co, 1982.

Nutrition

Herbert T. Cohen, M.D.

I. General concepts.

Hospitalized patients generally require nutritional support when they have been without oral intake for 5 days and are anticipated to continue so for another 7 days. In certain patients, early initiation of nutritional support seems advantageous, i.e., burn victims, and patients who may have a better prognosis with supplementation, i.e., patients with acute renal failure. Routes of administration include enteral: either oral or via a feeding tube; and parenteral: either via a peripheral or central vein. Generally, enteral feedings are preferable to parenteral because of their more physiologic metabolism and lower incidence of complications.

II. Calorie and protein requirements.

A. Unstressed patients, sedentary:
Kcals: 30 Kcal/kg body weight,
protein: 0.8 g/kg body weight.

B. Moderately stressed patients: postop, intensive care, ventilator dependent:
Kcals: 40 Kcal/kg,
protein: 0.8–1.2 g/kg.

C. Severely stressed: burn, multiple trauma victim:
Kcals: 60 Kcal/kg,
protein: 1.2–2.0 g/kg.
Caloric yields of dietary components:
carbohydrate = 4 Kcal/g;
protein = 4 Kcal/g;
fat = 9 Kcal/g.

III. Initiation of feedings.

A. General:

Determine calorie and protein requirements and calculate total volume of feeding desired per day.

If the volume is impractical, calories can be supplemented with fat.

B. Enteral:

Begin infusion with full strength at 20 mL per hour over 24 hours and increase rate of infusion 10 mL per hour per day to desired daily volume as tolerated.

C. Parenteral:

1. Central venous nutrition (CVN):

Day 1: 1 L D10W over 24 hours.

Day 2: 1 L CVN over 24 hours.

Subsequently increase daily volume as desired.

Supplement 500 mL of 10% or 20% Liposyn two to three times per week.

2. Peripheral venous nutrition (PVN):

Can begin PVN on day 1.

Can supplement daily with 500 mL of 10% Liposyn.

Simultaneous infusion of PVN and Liposyn via ''Y'' connection decreases osmolality of PVN infusion and can limit phlebitis.

Can supplement insulin for hyperglycemia. Administer trace elements, phosphorus, potassium, etc., as necessary.

IV. Monitoring/precautions.

A. General:

1. Avoid abrupt changes in rates of feedings to avoid hyperglycemia, hypertriglyceridemia, and rebound hypoglycemia.

2. To decrease carbon dioxide production, as when weaning from ventilator, avoid giving excess calories and provide high percentage (45% to 50%) of nonprotein calories as fat in place of carbohydrates.

   B. Enteral:
      1. Keep head of bed elevated >30°.
      2. Add methylene blue to monitor for aspiration.
      3. Check residual volume of feedings.
   C. Parenteral:
      1. Follow up electrolytes and glucose daily.
      2. Follow up liver chemistries, magnesium, calcium, phosphorus, two to three times per week.
      3. Use a single central port for CVN alone.
      4. Compare pre- and 8 to 10 hour postlipid infusion triglyceride levels. If twofold or greater increase is noted, hold lipid infusion.

V. Enteral feeding formulary.
   Can be used orally or via feeding tube:
   A. Nutritionally complete feeding (lactose base).
      1. Osmolyte (isotonic).
         a. 1.06 Kcal/mL.
         b. 37 g protein/L.
         c. 300 mOsm.
         d. 27 mEq Na^+; 26 mEq K^+.
      2. Ensure Plus.
         a. 1.5 Kcal/mL.
         b. 55 g protein/L.
         c. 600 mOsm.
         d. 50 mEq Na^+; 55 mEq K^+.
      3. Ensure enrich (13 g fiber/L).
         a. 1.1 Kcal/mL.
         b. 39 g protein/L.
         c. 480 mOsm.
         d. 36 mEq Na^+; 38 mEq K^+.
      4. Isocal HCN.
         a. 2 Kcal/mL.
         b. 75 g protein/L.
         c. 690 mOsm.
         d. 35 mEq Na^+; 43 mEq K^+.
   B. Elemental feedings (for malabsorption; absorbed in upper gut).
      1. Vital.

       a. 1 Kcal/mL.

       b. 42 g protein/L.

       c. 500 mOsm.

       d. 20 mEq Na$^+$; 34 mEq K$^+$.

   2. Vivonex.

       a. 1 Kcal/mL.

       b. 43 g protein/L.

       c. 810 mOsm.

       d. 23 mEq Na$^+$; 30 mEq K$^+$.

C. Special feedings.

   1. Aminaid (high in essential amino acids).

       a. 2 Kcal/mL.

       b. 19 g protein/L.

       c. 800 mOsm.

       d. 14 mEq Na$^+$; <5 mEq K$^+$.

   2. Hepatic aid (high in branched-chain amino acids).

       a. 1.6 Kcal/mL.

       b. 44 g protein/L.

       c. 570 mOsm.

       d. <14 mEq Na$^+$; <5 mEq K$^+$.

D. Modular feedings.

   1. Carbohydrate.

       a. Polycose.

           i. 2 Kcal/mL.

           ii. 500 g carbohydrate/L.

           iii. 850 mOsm.

           iv. 12 mEq Na$^+$; 2.6 mEq K$^+$.

   2. Protein.

       a. Propac powder (all protein).

           i. 4 Kcal/g.

           ii. 15 g protein/packet.

           iii. 45 mg Na$^+$/packet; 100 mg K$^+$/packet.

   3. Fat.

       a. MCT oil (for malabsorption; medium-chain triglycerides).

           i. 7.7 Kcal/mL.

       b. Microlipid (essential fatty acid supplement).

           i. 4.5 Kcal/mL.

VI. Parenteral feeding formulary.
  A. Standard CVN (2 U MVI, 1 U trace elements added by pharmacy daily).
    1. 1.01 cal/mL.
    2. 42.5 g protein/L.
    3. 1,850 mOsm.
    4. 35 mEq Na^+; 30 mEq K^+.
  B. Renal CVN (2 U MVI, 1 U trace elements added by pharmacy daily, no potassium, low protein as branched-chain amino acids).
    1. 1.34 cal/mL.
    2. 27 g protein/L.
    3. 2,000 mOsm.
    4. 20 mEq Na^+; 0 mEq K^+.
  C. Hepatic CVN (2 U MVI, 1 U trace elements added by pharmacy daily).
    1. 1.0 cal/mL.
    2. 40 g protein/L.
    3. 1,850 mOsm.
    4. 35 mEq Na^+; 30 mEq K^+.
  D. Standard PVN.
    1. 0.285 cal/mL.
    2. 27 g protein/L.
    3. 710 mOsm.
    4. 35 mEq Na^+; 30 mEq K^+.
VII. Fat supplements.
  A. 10% Liposyn.
    1. 550 kcal/500 mL dose.
    2. 300 mOsm.
  B. 20% Liposyn.
    1. 1,000 kcal/500 mL dose.
    2. 340 mOsm.
  C. Administration:
    Test dose: 1 mL/min for 15 to 30 minutes. If tolerated, continue over 4 to 6 hours.

Acknowledgment: Sally Wagner, M.S., R.D.

Formulary

13

James Lane, M.D.

TABLE 13–1.
Common Drugs

Drug	How Supplied	Dose	Comments
Acetaminophen (Tylenol)	325 mg tabs or caplets, 160 mg/5 mL children's elixir. Extra-strength available as 500 mg tabs or caplets and in elixir 1,000 mg per ounce. Suppositories: 120, 125, 130, 300, 325, 500, 600, 650 mg.	325 to 650 mg every 4 hr to a maximum of 4 g per day.	Effective analgesic and antipyretic. Has little antiinflammatory effect. May cause renal injury with excess use. Potentiates oral anticoagulants in large doses. May cause severe hepatic damage and death. Early symptoms include nausea, vomiting, diarrhea, diaphoresis, pallor, and abdominal pain. Acetylcysteine is drug of choice with overdose. Caution should be used in administering this to patients with liver disease.
Acetazolamide (Diamox)	Intravenous (IV): 500 mg vials. Orally (PO): 125 and 250 mg tabs.	IV: 250 mg two to three times per day. PO: 250 mg two to four times per day.	Used for pseudotumor cerebri and open angle glaucoma. Diuretic effects initially. Causes metabolic acidosis, anorexia, drowsiness, seizures, hypokalemia, rash, cytopenias, and hirsutism.
Acyclovir (Zovirax)	IV in 100 mL dextrose 5% in water (D5W) or normal saline (NS). PO: 200 mg tabs.	5–10 mg/kg every 8 hr IV. 200 mg PO 5 times per day.	Antiviral agent. Nephrotoxic. CNS side effects common. Reduce dose in renal disease. Herpes simplex use lower IV dose, except encephalitis. Zoster: use higher IV dose.

Albuterol (Ventolin, Proventil)	Metered dose inhaler. PO: 2 mg, 4 mg tabs.	Two puffs every 4–6 hrs and prn.	β-2 agonist. Action and side effects similar to metaproterenol.
Alprazolam (Xanax)	0.25 mg, 0.5 mg, 1.0 mg tabs	Starting dosage of 0.25–0.5 mg TID to max daily dosage of 4 mg.	Benzodiazepine. Mean t-1/2 of 12–15 hrs. Drowsiness is most common side effect but less than diazepam.
Amantadine (Symmetrel)	PO: 100 mg tab. Syrup: 10 mg/1 mL.	100 mg PO BID.	Antiviral agent. Prophylaxis of influenza A, including swine and Russian strains. Treatment of influenza A if in first 24 hours of illness. Also used in Parkinson's disease.
Amphotericin B (Fungizone)	IV diluted in D5W only.	0.25–0.5 mg/kg/day to a total dose determined by illness.	Antifungal agent. Give test dose 1 mg in D5W over at least 30 min, followed by 0.25 mg/kg over 4 hrs. Daily dose can be increased in 5–10 mg increments on each subsequent day. Can premedicate with acetaminophen, steroids, and/or antihistamines. Side effects: reversible nephrotoxicity, hypokalemia, hypomagnesemia, bone marow suppression, thrombophlebitis.

TABLE 13–1. *(cont.)*
Common Drugs

Drug	How Supplied	Dose	Comments
Amiodarone (Cordarone)	200 mg tabs.	PO loading dose: 800–1600 mg/day for 1–3 wks then 600–800 mg/day for 4 wks. PO maintenance dose: 100–400 mg/day.	Anti-arrhythmic. Long half-life (wks). Prolongs PR, QRS, and QT intervals. Side effects are bradycardia, heartblock, ventricular fibrillation or tachycardia, gastrointestinal (GI) upset, hepatitis, ataxia, tremor, dizziness, pulmonary fibrosis, corneal deposits, and hyper- or hypothyroidism. Effects may persist for months after drug is stopped.
Amoxicillin	PO: 250, 500 mg.	PO: 750–1500 mg/day; Interval: every 8 hrs.	Semi-synthetic penicillin. Lengthen interval when the creatinine clearance decreases. Rash more common than with other penicillins.
Amoxicillin and Clavulanic acid (Augmentin)	PO: 250, 500 mg capsules or oral suspension.	250–500 mg PO every 6–8 hrs.	Clavulanic acid broadens amoxicillin coverage to include β-lactamase organisms. Covers gram-positive (staph) and gram-negative bacteria (*Hemophilus influenza*), anaerobes.

Drug		Dose	
Amphotericin B (Fungizone)	IV diluted in D5W only.	0.25–0.5 mg/kg/day to a total dose determined by illness.	Antifungal agent. Give test dose 1 mg in D5W over at least 30 min, followed by 0.25 mg/kg over 4 hrs. Daily dose can be increased in 5–10 mg increments on each subsequent day. Can premedicate with acetaminophen, steroids, and/or antihistamines. Side effects: reversible nephrotoxicity, hypokalemia, hypomagnesemia, bone marow suppression, thrombophlebitis.
Ampicillin	PO: 250 and 500 mg. Also IV, IM. IV diluted in 50–100 mL NS or D5W.	PO: 1–4 g/day; IV/IM: 2–12 g/day; interval: every 6–8 hrs.	Synthetic penicillin. Lengthen interval when creatinine clearance decreases. Rash, diarrhea more common than with other penicillins. May decrease effect of oral contraceptives.
Amrinone (Inocor)	20 mL amps with 5 mg/l mL.	Loading dose 0.7 mg/kg over 2–3 min IV. Maintenance: 5–10 mcg/kg/min to total daily dose not to exceed 10 mg/kg.	Inotropic agent. Side effects are GI upset, hepatoxicity, thrombocytopenia, myalgias, fever, and ventricular irritability.

TABLE 13–1. (cont.)
Common Drugs

Drug	How Supplied	Dose	Comments
Antacids (Mylanta II)	Liquid suspension or tabs.	Liquid: 30 mL PO between meals and at bedtime. Tabs: 2 tab PO between meals and at bedtime.	Balanced formula of aluminum and magnesium minimizes diarrhea and constipation. Used only with caution in renal failure.
(Alternagel, Amphogel)	Liquid suspension or tabs.	Same as above.	May cause constipation.
Aspirin	Available as tabs and suppositories. Plain tabs: 325 mg; enteric coated tabs: 325 mg, 650 mg.	Dosage variable depending on indication.	Antinflammatory agent. Will prolong the bleeding time 4–7 days after a single dose. Used in patients with coronary artery disease, cerebrovascular disease, prosthetic valves, and for its analgesic, antipyretic and antiinflammatory properties. Contraindications similar to heparin. Complications include hemorrhage, gastritis, peptic ulcer disease, and salicylate intoxication.
Atenolol (Tenormin)	50 and 100 mg tabs.	50–100 mg PO daily, given once a day.	β-receptor antagonist. β-1 selective with hydrophilic properties.

Atropine	Available for use with a nebulizer.	2–4 mg with nebulizer every 4–6 hrs.	Onset of activity is 15–30 min. Peak effect in 1–3 hrs. Major side effect is dry mouth.
Atropine	1 mg in 10 mL syringe.	0.5–1.0 mg every 5 hrs up to 2.0 mg total.	Does less than 0.5 mg may cause paradoxical vagotonic effect.
Azlocillin (Azlin)	IV diluted in 100 mL D5W or NS.	IV: 18 g/day at dose of 3 g every 4 hrs.	Extended-spectrum penicillin. Increase creatinine clearance decreases. Platelet dysfunction, hypokalemia.
Aztreonam (Azactam)	IV diluted in 50–100 mL D5W or NS.	1–2 g every 8 hrs.	Monobactam antibiotic. Aerobic gram-negative bacteria coverage. No known crossreactivity with penicillins.
Beclomethasone (Vanceril, Beclovent)	Metered dose inhaler.	Two puffs every 4–6 hrs.	Inhaled steroids. Benefit in decreasing or eliminating the need for oral steroids. May cause oral thrush.
Bretylium (Bretylol)	500 mg in 10 mL syringe for IV push. Diluted for IV infusion.	Loading dose: 5 mg/kg IV with subsequent dose of 10 mg/kg to a maximum of 30 mg/kg. Maintenance dose: 1–4 mg/min IV infusion.	Anti-arrhythmic. Side effects are hypotension, nausea, vomiting. Increases the heart's sensitivity to catecholamines. Bretylium may initially worsen arrhythmias.

TABLE 13–1. (cont.)
Common Drugs

Drug	How Supplied	Dose	Comments
Bromocriptine	PO: 2.5 mg tabs and 5.0 mg capsules.	1.25 mg PO BID as initial dose, may be increased 2.5 mg/day every 2–4 wks until response achieved.	Dopamine agonist used in Parkinson's disease. Causes nausea, vomiting, abnormal involuntary movements, hallucinations, ataxia, insomnia, depression, anorexia, anxiety, dry mouth, edema of lower extremities, incontinence, and muscle cramps. May elevate the BUN, SGOT, SGPT, CPK, and alkaline phosphatase levels.
Calcitonin (Calcimar)	400 IU/2mL for subcutaneous (SQ) use.	4 U/kg BID, 8 U/kg QID.	Used as therapy in Paget's disease and hypercalcemia. Common adverse reactions are nausea, vomiting, and local inflammation at site of injection. Decreased efficacy after several days use.
Calcitriol (Rocaltrol)	0.25 and 0.50 mcg capsules.	0.25–1.0 mcg per day.	The most active vitamin D metabolite. It has a rapid onset and a short half-life. Calcitriol is especially effective in severe renal failure.

Calcium carbonate (Os-Cal 500)	Each tablet with 500 mg elemental calcium.	2–4 tabs PO daily (1–2 g elemental calcium per day).	Well absorbed unless stomach non-acidic.
Calcium chloride	10% solution in 10 mL syringe for IV use.	5–10 mL IV as needed, with rate not to exceed 1 mL/min.	Three times more calcium than any other preparation. Drug of choice in severe hypocalcemia. Very irritating to subcutaneous tissues and veins.
Calcium gluconate	IV: 10% solution in 10 mL containers. PO: 500 mg tab available generically.	IV: 20 mL of 10% solution given slowly. May be given as continuous infusion. PO: 15 g daily in divided doses.	Contains 9% elemental calcium. Nonirritating to veins. IV calcium should be administered carefully to patients receiving digoxin.
Captopril (Capoten)	12.5, 25, 50, and 100 mg tabs.	6.25–25 mg PO TID.	Angiotensin-coverting enzyme inhibitor. May cause hypotension, neutropenia, rash, dysgeusia, proteinuria, and renal insufficiency.
Carbenicillin (Geopen)	IM, IV: IV diluted in 50 mL D5W or NS.	For severe infections: 400–600 mg/kg/day, interval: every 4–6 hrs.	Extended spectrum penicillin. Hypokalemia/hypernatremia, transaminitis, coagulopathy.

TABLE 13-1. *(cont.)*
Common Drugs

Drug	How Supplied	Dose	Comments
Cefamandole (Mandol)	IM, IV diluted in 100 mL D5W or NS.	0.5–2.0 g, every 4–6 hrs, IV or IM.	Second generation cephalosporin. Gram-positive bacteria (not enterocococci; methicillin-resistant staph), gram-negative bacteria (not *Pseudomonas, Serratia*). Anaerobes (not *Bacteroides fragilis*).
Cefotaxime (Claforan)	IM, IV diluted in 100 ml D5W or NS.	1.0 g every 6 hours to 2.0 g every 4 hours IV or IM.	Third generation cephalosporin. Less gram-positive coverage then cefamandole, but better gram-negative coverage. Treats few *Pseudomonas.* Treats β-lactamase producing *H. influenza.* Crosses CSF.
Cefoxitin (Mefoxin)	IM, IV diluted in 50 mL D5W or NS.	1.0 g every 8 hours to 2.0 g every 4 hours IV or IM.	Second generation cephalosporin. Gram-positive (not enterococci; methicillin-resistant staphylococci), gram-negative (not *Pseudomonas, Enterobacter*). Anaerobes, including *B. fragilis.* May induce β-lactamases.

Drug	Preparation	Dose	Comments
Ceftazidime (Fortaz, Tazidime, Tazicef)	IM, IV diluted in 100 mL D5W or NS.	1.0–2.0 g every 8–12 hrs IV or IM.	Third generation cephalosporin. Effective against gram-positive bacteria (but less active than cefotaxime), gram-negative bacteria, including *Enterobacter*, *Pseudomonas*, anaerobes (not *B. fragilis*).
Ceftriaxone (Rocephin)	IM, IV diluted in 100 mL D5W or NS.	1.0–2.0 g every 24 hrs (may be given every 12 hrs, with total daily dose not to exceed 4 g).	Third generation cephalosporin with minimal *Pseudomonas* activity. Effective against gonorrheal infections. Crosses CSF.
Cephalexin (Keflex)	PO: 250 and 500 mg capsules or oral suspension.	PO: 250–500 mg every 6 hrs.	First generation cephalosporin. Effective against gram-positive bacteria (not enterococci), gram-negative (not *Enterobacter*, *Pseudomonas*, *Acinetobacter*). 9% eosinophilia.
Cephalothin (Keflin)	IM, IV diluted in 50 mL D5W or NS.	0.5–2.0 g every 4 to 6 hrs IV or IM.	First generation cephalosporin. Coverage similar to cephalexin. Phlebitis, pain on IM injection.
Chloramphenicol (Chloromycetin)	IV, PO: 250 mg IV diluted in 50 mL D5W or NS.	250–750 mg every 6 hrs.	Antibiotic. Broad coverage of many gram-positive and gram-negative bacteria, anaerobes, rarely can cause aplastic anemia.

TABLE 13–1. (cont.)
Common Drugs

Drug	How Supplied	Dose	Comments
Chlordiazepoxide (Librium)	5 mg, 10 mg, 25 mg capsules. IV, IM in 100 mg amps.	Anxiety: 5–25 mg PO TID-QID; ethanol withdrawal: 25–100 mg PO, IM, or IV QID. May repeat every 20 min up to 300 mg/24 hrs.	t-1/2 of 24–48 hrs. Lower dosages should be used for mild symptoms in the elderly. Less potent than valium on a milligram basis with less anticonvulsant and muscle relaxant properties; similar side effects as valium.
Chlorpheniramine maleate (Chlor-Trimeton)	4 mg tabs, timed-release tablets of 8 mg, 12 mg.	4 mg QID; 8–12 mg BID for timed-release formulation.	Has maximum therapy/sedation ratio, but still mildly sedative. Common ingredient in cold remedies.
Cholestyramine (Questran)	4 g powder packets.	16–24 g/day. Given QID.	Used in therapy for hypercholesterolemia and pruritus associated with biliary obstruction. Causes constipation, abdominal discomfort, nausea, vomiting, flatulence, and anorexia. Prevents absorption of many drugs and fat-soluble vitamins. May cause steatorrhea, bleeding tendency, and night blindness.

Cimetidine (Tagamet)	PO: 200, 300, 400, 800 mg tabs, 300 mg/5 mL liquid. Parenteral: 300 mg/2 mL diluted in 100 mL D5W or NS.	400 mg PO BID for active ulcer disease. 400 mg PO at bedtime for ulcer prophylaxis. Higher doses may be necessary in Zollinger-Ellison syndrome.	Inhibits H2 receptors with decrease in gastric acidity. May cause diarrhea, confusion, gynecomastia, impotence, thrombocytopenia, and neutropenia. Decrease dose and interval in renal failure.
Clindamycin (Cleocin)	PO: 75, 100 mg tabs. IM, IV diluted in 50–100 mL D5W or NS.	PO: 150–300 mg PO every 6 hrs. IV: 150–900 mg IV every 6 hrs.	Semisynthetic lincomycin antibiotic. Anaerobic bacteria, and susceptible strep and staph. No adjustment necessary for renal failure. Can produce pseudomembranous colitis.
Clofibrate (Atromid-S)	500 mg capsules.	500 mg TID to QID.	Used as therapy for primary dysbetalipoproteinemia and hypertriglyceridemia. Has little effect on hypercholesterolemia. Causes nausea, vomiting, loose stools, flatulence, and abdominal distress. Contraindicated in pregnancy, renal disease, and hepatic disease. May have increased mortality after a myocardial infarction.

TABLE 13–1. *(cont.)*
Common Drugs

Drug	How Supplied	Dose	Comments
Clonidine (Catapres)	PO: 0.1, 0.2, 0.3 mg tabs; transdermal patches: 0.1, 0.2, 0.3 mg patches.	0.1–2.0 mg PO BID or TID. 0.2 mg PO followed by 0.1 mg/hr up to 0.7 mg total for accelerating hypertension. Use patch weekly.	Centrally acting antihypertensive. Common adverse effects are drowsiness, dry mouth, constipation, depression, impotence, and the rebound phenomenon on withdrawal of the medication.
Cyproheptadine (Periactin)	4 mg tabs; 2 mg/5 mL syrup.	2–4 mg PO QID.	Antihistamine. Used in treatment of migraine and cluster headaches. Causes drowsiness and dry mouth. Contraindicated with monoamine oxidase inhibitors and in glaucoma.
Dantrolene sodium (Dantrium)	IV: 70 mL vials with 20 mg dantrolene and 3,000 mg mannitol. PO: 25, 50, 100 mg capsules.	For malignant hyperthermia: 1 mg/kg by IV push. Should continue until symptoms subside or total dose of 10 mg/kg is reached. PO: 4–8 mg/kg/day in four divided doses.	Useful for the spasticity of upper motor neuron disorders. Also used emergently for neuroleptic malignant syndrome. It produces weakness, drowsiness, dizziness, nausea, vomiting, and diarrhea. Most serious adverse reaction is hepatoxicity. Use in active liver disease contraindicated.

Desferoxamine (Desferal)	Vials of 500 mg for IM/SQ/ IV administration. IM is preferred route.	Acute iron intoxication: 1 g IM then 500 mg IM every 4 hrs twice; after initial dose, may give 500 mg IM every 4–12 hrs, not to exceed 6 g/ 24 hrs. Nonemergent: 1–2 g continuous IV infusion or subcutaneous or 0.5–1 g IM every day; 2 g IV with each unit transfused.	Indicated for iron overload states, transfusion-dependent anemia such as severe sideroblastic anemia and thalassemia, hemochromatosis when severe anemia precludes phlebotomy. Side effects: anaphylaxis, local soreness and erythema at injured site, rarely cataracts.
Dexamethasone (Decadron)	PO: 0.50, 0.75, 1.5, 4 mg tabs; elixir: 0.5 mg/5 mL. Parenteral: 4 mg/ mL, 10 mg/mL.	10 mg IV push initially. Followed by 4 mg every 6 hrs. PO: 4 mg every 6 hrs and taper to maintenance dose.	Associated with all the hazards of glucocorticoids. To be avoided in patients with systemic infections. High doses associated with peptic ulcer disease. Causes hypokalemia, salt and water retention, myopathy, osteoporosis, hyperglycemia.

TABLE 13-1. *(cont.)*
Common Drugs

Drug	How Supplied	Dose	Comments
Diazepam (Valium)	2 mg, 5 mg, 10 mg tabs. Parenteral: 10 mg/2 mL vials.	Anxiety: 2–10 mg PO, IM or IV BID or QID; ethanol withdrawal: 5–10 mg IM or IV, repeated in 3–4 hrs if needed; seizure control (should not be used as sole therapy): 5–10 mg IM or IV initially; may repeat at 10–15 min intervals to max dose of 30 mg. Not to be infused faster than 5 mg 5 mg/min/min.	Benzodiazepine. t-1/2 averages 30 hrs. Side effects: drowsiness, fatigue, ataxia, blurred vision, hypotension, paradoxical excitement, thrombophlebitis at injection site.
Dicloxacillin (Dynapen)	PO: 250, 500 mg.	PO: 0.5–2 g/day; interval: every 6 hrs.	No change for renal insufficiency. Associated with GI bleeding.
Digoxin (Lanoxin)	PO: 0.125 mg, 0.25 mg tabs. IV: 0.5 mg/2 mL amps.	Maintenance dose is 0.125–0.25/day, may use loading dose of 0.5–1.0 mg.	Cardiac glycoside. Quinidine, verapamil, and amiodarone increase serum levels. Usual serum levels are 0.5–2.0 mg/mL. Toxicities are atrioventricular block, dysrhythmia, nausea, blurred or yellow vision, and gynecomastia. Dysrhythmias are worse in the presence of hypokalemia and/or hypercalcemia.

Drug	Supply	Dose	Comments
Diltiazem (Cardizem)	30 and 60 mg tabs.	120–360 mg/day given PO every 6–8 hrs.	Calcium channel blocker with least amount of vasodilation. Affects atrioventricular nodal conduction.
Diphenhydramine (Benadryl)	25 and 50 mg capsules, 12.5 mg/5 mL elixir; parenteral: 10 mg/mL for IM/IV use.	25–50 mg QID.	Antihistamine. Highly sedative. May mask the ototoxicity of ototoxic antibiotics.
Dipyridamole (Persantine)	25, 50, 75 mg tabs.	150–400 mg per day in three doses.	It is a coronary vasodilator and may inhibit platelet cyclic nucleotide phosphodiesterase. May cause GI upset.
Disopyramide (Norpace)	100, 150 mg capsules.	Load: 4 mg/kg PO. Maintenance: 100–200 mg Q8°.	Antiarrhythmic. Prolongs QRS, QT ($\pm$ PR) intervals. Anticholinergic, negative inotrope, hepatic toxicity, psychosis, agranulocytosis.
Dobutamine (Dobutrex)	250 mg/20 mL vial. Must be further diluted with at least 50 mL D5W.	2–20 mcg/kg/min IV.	Increases cardiac contractility and is a mild vasodilator. Contraindicated in idiopathic hypertrophic subaortic stenosis.
Dopamine (Intropin)	Diluted for IV use. Common concentration: 800 mg/250 mL.	2–20 mcg/kg/min IV.	< 5 mcg/kg/min causes selective mesenteric and renal vasodilatation, 2–5 mcg/kg/min for renal perfusion. 5–10 mcg/kg/min is inotropic. > 10 mcg/kg/min causes vasoconstriction.

TABLE 13–1. *(cont.)*
Common Drugs

Drug	How Supplied	Dose	Comments
Edrophonium (Tensilon)	10 mL and 1 mL ampuls at 10 mg/mL.	Test dose for myasthenia gravis: 2 mg IV push over 30 sec. If no reaction after 45 sec give remaining 8 mg; myasthenic crisis: 1 mg IV initially. If no improvement after 1 min give second IV dose.	Rapid-acting cholinergic drug. A positive response for myasthenia gravis is increased muscle strength without fasciculations. Brief duration of action. Not recommended for maintenance therapy. Contraindicated in patients with intestinal or urinary obstruction. Atropine should be available when doing this maneuver. Side effects are bradycardia, miosis, lacrimation, convulsions, dysphagia, respiratory paralysis, bronchoconstriction, diaphoresis, and muscle weakness. Cholinergic response often seen in myasthenics who have been overtreated with anticholinesterase drugs.
Enalapril (Vasotec)	5 and 10 mg tabs.	5–40 mg PO daily in one dose.	Angiotensin-converting enzyme inhibitor.
Epinephrine	Suspension 1:1,000 in 1 and 2 mL containers (1 mg/mL).	SQ: 0.3–0.5 mg prn to 1 mg in 2 hrs or 2 mg in 24 hrs.	Onset of action is 1–3 min. Peak effect in 15–20 min. Side effects include tremors and tachycardia. May precipitate cardiac ischemia in patients at risk.

		1 mL amp (1 mg in 1:1,000 dilution). 10 mL syringe (1 mg in 1:10,000 dilution).	0.5–1 mg IV push every 5 min or 1–4 mcg/min continuous IV infusion.	α- and β-agonist. Useful in cardiac arrest for treatment of ventricular fibrillation, electromechanical dissociation, and hypotension.
Ergocalciferol (vitamin D2)	50,000 unit capsules, drops: 8,000 U/mL, injection 500,000 U/mL.	40,000–100,000 U per day.	Used to treat hypoparathyroidism, rickets, and osteomalacia associated with hypophosphatemia and renal tubular disorders. There is a lag of 10–14 days between the initiation of therapy and a therapeutic effect.
Ergotamine preparations (Cafergot)	Each tablet with 1 mg ergotamine and 100 mg caffeine. Suppositories with 2 mg ergotamine and 100 mg caffeine.	PO: 2 tabs at onset of migraine. An additional tab can be taken every 30 min to total of 6 tabs/ day or 10 tabs/wk. Rectally: 1 suppository at onset and another after 1 hr. Maximum of 2/attack and 5/wk.	Aborts or prevents vascular headaches. Contraindicated in renal failure, hepatic failure, angina, peripheral vascular disease, pregnancy, and hypertension. Causes nausea and vomiting, numbness, tingling, and cramps. Mental status changes rare.
Erythromycin	Parenteral: 500–1,000 mg vials diluted in 250 mL NS or D5W.	500–1,000 mg every 6 hrs IV; PO: 250–500 mg every 6 hr. May add 10 mg lidocaine to IV form to decrease pain at injection site.	Effective against gram-positive bacteria, Legionnella, mycoplasma. Nausea common, phlebitis common. Ototoxic at higher doses.

TABLE 13–1. *(cont.)*
Common Drugs

Drug	How Supplied	Dose	Comments
Ethambutol (Myambutol)	PO: 100 mg, 400 mg tabs.	15 mg/kg as a single oral dose once every 24 hrs.	Bacteriostatic to both extracellular and intracellular mycobacterium tuberculosis. Can cause optic neuritis with decreased visual acuity, central scotomata and red-green color blindness. Monitor visual acuity.
Ethacrynic acid (Edecrin)	IV: supplied in vials of 50 mg; PO: 25 and 50 mg tabs.	IV: 50–100 mg as needed. PO: 25–200 mg every day.	Loop diuretic. Similar to furosemide, but higher incidence of ototoxicity.
Ethosuximide (Zarontin)	PO: 250 mg capsules and 250 mg/5 mL syrup.	Initial dose 500 mg/day. Increased by 250 mg every 4–7 days. Given two to three times per day for daily dose > 1000 mg.	Given for petit mal seizures. Causes nausea, vomiting, anorexia, drowsiness, headache, dizziness, euphoria, hiccups, rash.
Etidronate disodium (Didronel)	200 mg tabs.	5–20 mg/kg every day PO.	Indicated for long-term treatment of Paget's disease. Should not be used for longer than 6 mo continuously. Most common adverse reactions are hypersensitivity reactions.

Famotidine (Pepcid)	PO: 20, 40 mg tabs and oral suspension 40 mg/5 mL; IV: 10 mg/mL.	For active ulcers 40 mg at bedtime or 20 mg BID. For maintenance, 20 mg at bedtime.	H2 antagonist for peptic ulcer disease. Headache in 5%. Decrease dose and interval in severe renal disease. No known drug interactions.
Ferrous sulfate	300 mg tabs 60 mg elemental iron. Elixir: 300 mg/5 mL.	Sufficient to provide between 150–200 mg elemental iron daily in three or four divided doses 1 hr before meals.	Side effects: mainly GI complaints including nausea, constipation, diarrhea, abdominal cramping. Over the counter preparations adequate as long as ferrous form and non-enteric coated.
Flecainide (Tambocor)	100 mg tabs.	100 mg BID, then increase by 50 mg every 12 hrs every 4–6 days as needed up to 400 mg/day.	Anti-arrhythmic. Prolongs PR/QRS, bradycardia, atrioventricular block, negative inotrope, GI upset, CNS effects. Can be pro-arrhythmic.
Flurazepam (Dalmane)	15 mg, 30 mg capsules.	15–30 mg at bedtime.	Hypnotic. Long t-1/2 of 24–100 hrs. Rebound insomnia less than with shorter-acting benzodiazepines but daytime somnolence may be a problem, especially in the elderly.

TABLE 13–1. *(cont.)*
Common Drugs

Drug	How Supplied	Dose	Comments
Folic acid	1 mg tabs, 5 mg/mL vial in 10 mL multi-dose vials.	1–5 mg PO every day.	Minimum daily requirement of 50 g. May improve GI and hematologic abnormalities of B12 deficiency while neurologic symptoms may progress. Ubiquitous in green vegetables, liver, kidneys.
Furosemide (Lasix)	IV: 10 mg/mL in vials and prefilled syringes. PO: 20, 40, 80 mg tabs.	IV: 20–80 mg as needed. PO: 40–80 mg once or twice a day.	Loop diuretic. GI side effects include anorexia, nausea, vomiting, abdominal cramps, and pancreatitis. May cause tinnitus and hearing loss. Other effects include cytopenias, rash, photosensitivity, hyperuricemia, hypernatremia, hypokalemia, and hypocalcemia. May precipitate lithium toxicity.
Gemfibrozil (Lopid)	300 mg capsules.	600 mg PO BID.	Lipid lowering agent. Similar to clofibrate. Associated with increased high density lipoprotein (HDL)-cholesterol.

Gentamicin (Garamycin)	IV, IM 2 mL = 80 mg vial. Diluted in 100 mL D5W or NS.	1.5 mg/kg every 8 hrs.	Aminoglycoside antibiotic. Effective against aerobic gram-negative bacteria, staphylococci. Nephrotoxic, ototoxic. Loading dose the same in renal disease, but then must increase interval and follow-up pre- and post-dose levels. Pre-dose less than 2, 1 hr postinfusion, 4–10 mg/ml.
Haloperidol (Haldol)	0.5 mg, 1 mg, 2 mg, 5 mg, 10 mg, 20 mg tabs. Parenteral: 1 mL = 5 mg.	0.5–5 mg PO BID or TID. Acute agitation: 2–5 mg IM, administered hourly if needed. with daily dosage as high as 100 mg.	Tranquilizer. Increased dosages may be needed for severe symptoms; lower initial dosages should be used for the elderly. Relatively nonsedating, but side effects include extrapyramidal reactions, usually dose-related, decreased blood pressure, tardive dyskinesia, neuroleptic malignant syndrome, dry mouth, blurred vision, urinary retention, and increased transaminases.

TABLE 13–1. (cont.)
Common Drugs

Drug	How Supplied	Dose	Comments
Heparin	Parenteral form, available as porcine or bovine preparations.	Prophylaxis: 5,000 SQ every 8–12 hrs; full anticoagulation: 10–20,000 U SQ initially and then 8–10,000 U every 8 hrs adjusted to partial thromboplastin time (PTT) or 5,000-U load followed by 18–30,000 U/24 hrs as continuous drip and adjusted to PTT.	Used in the treatment of venous and arterial thromboembolic disease. Contraindicated in peptic ulcer disease, malignant hypertension, hemorrhagic diatheses, recent surgical procedures, and brain tumors. Heparin accelerates the inhibitory activity of antithrombin III. Complications include hemorrhage, thrombocytopenia, osteoporosis (with chronic use of > 10,000/day), and elevated SGOT, SGPT. Use PTT to monitor therapy. Monitoring is essential to prevent hemorrhagic complications. Hematuria, melena, menorrhagia, petechiae, and gingival bleeding should prompt re-evaluation of the therapy.
Hydralazine (Apresoline)	PO: 10, 25, 50, 100 mg tabs; parenteral: 20 mg/mL amp.	40–300 mg PO/day in three or four doses. 10–20 mg IM or IV every 30 min.	Acts as a vasodilator. Causes reflex tachycardia. Lupus-like syndrome occurs in 10% to 15% with high doses (400 mg every day).

Hydrochlorothiazide (Esidrix, Hydrodiuril)	25, 50 mg tabs.	Usual dose, 50–100 mg PO once or twice a day.	Thiazide diuretic. Side effects include hyperglycemia, elevated uric acid, hypercalcemia, hyponatremia, hypokalemia, rash, photosensitivity, and cytopenias.
Hydroxyzine (Vistaril, Atarax)	Parenteral: 25 or 50 mg/mL for Vistaril IM use. PO: 10, 25, mg tabs and 10 mg/5 mL syrup for Atarax.	10–50 mg QID.	Useful in pruritic skin disease. Also helpful as anti-anxiety agent. Drowsiness most common reaction. Contraindicated during early pregnancy.
Ibuprofen (Motrin)	300, 400, 600, 800 mg tabs.	400 mg PO every 4–6 hrs.	May cause nausea, diarrhea, peptic ulcer disease, and abdominal cramping. Dizziness and headaches most common CNS effects. May cause edema secondary to sodium retention. May induce renal insufficiency, acute interstitial nephritis, hematuria, proteinuria, and the nephrotic syndrome. Contraindicated in patients with the syndrome of nasal polyps, angioedema, and bronchospastic reactivity to aspirin.

TABLE 13–1. (cont.)
Common Drugs

Drug	How Supplied	Dose	Comments
Imipenem + cilastatin (Primaxin)	IV only, diluted in 100–250 mL NS.	250–1,000 mg every 6 hrs.	Broad-spectrum antibiotic. Broad gram-positive, gram-negative, and anaerobic coverage, but inactive against methicillin-resistant staphylococci. Seizures can occur. Decrease dose in renal disease.
Indomethacin (Indocin)	25, 50, 75 mg capsules, 75 mg sustained release capsules; 25 mg/5 mL oral suspension; 50 mg suppositories.	50 mg PO TID. Sustained release preparation given 75 mg PO BID. Dosage not to exceed 200 mg/day.	Contraindicated in patients with history of asthma precipitated by aspirin. Suppositories contraindicated in patients with proctitis or recent rectal bleeding. Oral preparations should be given with food or antacids. May cause GI tract ulcerations and bleeding. As with other nonsteroidal antiinflammatory agents, prostaglandin inhibition will interfere with renal blood flow autoregulation and induce renal insufficiency in susceptible patients. May also cause acute tubulointerstitial disease, minimal change disease leading to nephrotic syndrome, sodium retention, and an antikaliuretic effect. Corneal deposits and retinal defects occur with pro-

		longed use. CNS effects include drowsiness, vertigo, headache, and tinnitus.
Ipratropium bromide (Atrovent)	2 puffs every 4–6 hrs.	Anticholinergic action for chronic obstructive pulmonary disease. Onset of action is 3–5 min. Duration of action is 3–6 hrs. Advantage: very little systemic effect.
Isoetharine (Bronkosol)	1% solution for nebulizer. 0.5 mL per medicated nebulizer every 4–6 hrs.	Onset of action is 1–3 min with peak effect at 5-15 min. Total duration of action is 30–60 min.
Isoniazid	PO: 50, 100, 300 mg tabs; injection: 100 mg/mL. 5–10 mg/kg/day up to 300 mg/day as 1 dose; usual adult dose is 300 mg/day.	Bactericidal to both extracellular and intracellular mycobacterium tuberculosis organisms; 10% of patients develop increased SGOT. Risk of INH hepatitis increases with age and alcohol intake. Stop drug if transaminases greater than four times normal. Must give with pyridoxine to prevent peripheral neuropathy.
Isoproterenol (Isuprel)	1 mg vials, diluted for IV infusion. Dilutions range from 4–6 mg/250 mL. 2–20 mcg/min.	Pure beta-agonist. Increases contractility and heart rate, and decreases peripheral resistance. May be arrhythmogenic. Increased myocardial oxygen demand.

TABLE 13-1. (cont.)
Common Drugs

Drug	How Supplied	Dose	Comments
Isosorbide dinitrate or trinitrate (Isordil)	Sublingual: 2.5, 5.0, and 10 mg tabs.	2.5–10 mg every 3–4 hrs.	Similar to nitroglycerin.
	Oral: 5, 10, 20 tabs.	20–60 mg PO every 6 hrs.	
	Sustained release: 40 mg tabs.	40–80 mg PO every 8–12 hrs.	
Ketoconazole (Nizoral)	PO: 200 mg tabs.	200–800 mg every day.	Antifungal agent. Dose-dependent nausea, decreased testosterone production, adrenal insufficiency, mild hepatotoxicity. Absorption dependent on gastric acidity.
Labetolol (Trandate, Normodyne)	PO: 100, 200, 300 mg tabs. IV: 100 mg/20 mL amps diluted for IV infusion. Usual dilution: 1 mg/mL.	200–1,200 mg PO/day, given every 12 hrs; 20–80 mg IV every 10 min up to 300 mg or 2 mg/min by continuous infusion.	It is both an α- and a β-blocker. Useful for accelerated hypertension.

Lactulose (Chronulac)	10 g/15 mL, 20 g/30 mL.	PO: 30 mL PO to titrate to a bowel movement every 8 hrs. Enema: 300 mL lactulose with 700 mL water or saline retained for 30–60 min. Repeat every 4–6 hrs PRN.	A poorly absorbable disaccharide which causes an osmotic diarrhea.
Levodopa with carbidopa (Sinemet)	PO: 10/100, 25/100, 25/250 tabs, (carbidopa/levodopa).	Daily dose must be titrated. Initial dose of 25/100 PO TID may be increased to six 25/100 tabs per day.	Carbidopa is a dopa decarboxylase inhibitor which prevents the extracerebral metabolism of levodopa. Side effects usually caused by levodopa include nausea, emesis, dyskinesia, psychiatric disturbances, postural hypotension. Should not be given with monoamine oxidase inhibitors. Seizures have occurred. Causes positive test for urine ketones. Patients with open angle glaucoma should have intraocular pressures monitored. Rarely causes anemia, leukopenia, and thrombocytopenia.

TABLE 13-1. (cont.)
Common Drugs

Drug	How Supplied	Dose	Comments
Levothyroxine (Synthroid)	Tabs of 25 mcg, 75 mcg, 100 mcg, 125 mcg, 150 mcg, 200 mcg, and 300 mcg. IV form also available as 500 mcg/5 mL.	25–150 mcg given once a day.	Thyroid replacement in the elderly requires a low dose and cautious incremental increases to avoid cardiac side effects. An IV form is available and is necessary for the treatment of myxedema coma. Suppression of TSH is a reliable indicator of adequate therapy.
Lidocaine (Xylocaine)	100 mg/10 mL syringe, 1 g/25 mL vial. Dilution for IV infusion: 2 g/250 mL.	Load: 1 mg/kg over 2 min, then 0.5 mg/kg over 10–20 min. Maintenance dose: 1–4 mg/min.	Anti-arrhythmic. May cause drowsiness, disorientation, coma, and seizures.
Lorazepam (Ativan)	0.5 mg, 1 mg, 2 mg tabs. Parenteral: 2 or 4 mg/mL in 1 mL and 10 mL vials.	Daily dosage of 1–10 mg orally (usually 2–6 mg).	Benzodiazepine. Short t-1/2 of 15 hrs, good oral and intramuscular absorption. May cause sedation, dizziness, disorientation, and hypotension.
Magnesium oxide	250 mg tabs.	1–2 g per day PO.	Causes diarrhea; contained in commercial antacids. Chronic therapy should be based on lab data.

Magnesium sulfate	Available for parenteral administration 1 g (8 meq) per 2 mL.	2–4 g IM or IV per day.	Used for magnesium depletion and in eclampsia. Replacement should be based on serum magnesium level.
Mannitol	Vial: 12.5 g/50 mL, 100 g/ 500 mL.	IV: give 1.0–1.5 mg/kg of the 20% solution over 10–30 min. May be repeated every 12 hrs.	Effects seen immediately. May cause hyperosmolar state. Aim for serum osmolality of 300–320 mOsm/L. It is an osmotic diuretic. Used to acutely decrease intracranial pressure and to reduce intraocular pressure prior to ocular surgery. Promotes urinary excretion of toxic substances. Hypernatremia common. May increase cerebral blood flow and worsen bleeding in neurosurgical patients.
Meclizine (Antivert)	PO: tabs 12.5, 25 mg.	25–100 mg PO in divided doses.	Antihistamine. Associated with drowsiness. Anticholinergic effect may worsen asthma or glaucoma. Other side effects include dry mouth and blurred vision.
Metaproterenol (Alupent)	Available for use in a nebulizer and by metered dose inhaler.	Nebulized, 0.3 mL in 3 mL NS every 3–4 hrs, metered dose inhaler 2 puffs every 4–6 hrs and PRN.	Onset of action within 3–6 min with peak effect at 20–60 min. Inhaled bronchodilators with fewer systemic side effects.

TABLE 13–1. *(cont.)*
Common Drugs

Drug	How Supplied	Dose	Comments
Methimazole	5 mg tabs.	Initial dose of 15–60 mg every 6 hrs for control of symptoms. Usual maintenance dose is 10–30 mg in two or three doses.	Does not inhibit peripheral conversion of T4 to T3. Adverse reactions similar to PTU. Can be crushed and given as rectal suppository in the obtunded patient with thyroid storm.
Methyldopa (Aldomet)	PO: 125, 250, 500 mg tabs, 250 mg/5 mL oral suspension. Parenteral: 250 mg/5 mL diluted in 100 mL D5W or NS.	500–2,000 mg/day given in two or three doses.	Anti-hypertensive. Side effects are drowsiness, dry mouth, nausea, vomiting, diarrhea, impotence, postural hypotension, and sodium and water retention. Hepatitis may occur and is reversible with discontinuation. Re-exposure to methyldopa may cause fatal hepatic necrosis. Twenty percent develop a positive Coomb's test but < 1% have hemolytic anemia.
Methysergide (Sansert)	2 mg tabs.	4–8 mg PO daily with meals.	Serotonin antagonist. Contraindicated in pregnancy, collagen vascular disease, renal disease, valvular disease, pulmonary disease, hepatic disease, peripheral vascular dis-

Methicillin (Staphcillin)	IM, IV diluted in 100 mL D5W or NS.	IM/IV: 6–12 g/day every 4–6 hrs.	Staphylococcal penicillin. Increase interval when creatinine clearance decreases. Hemorrhagic cystitis, platelet dysfunction, thrombocytopenia, nephropathy.

ease, hypertension, and coronary artery disease. Causes retroperitoneal, valvular, and pulmonary fibrosis. Other side effects include nausea, vomiting, vasoconstriction, and peripheral edema. Fibrosis reversible with discontinuation of drug. One mo off drug every 6 mo may prevent serious complications.

Methicillin (Staphcillin)	IM, IV diluted in 100 mL D5W or NS.	IM/IV: 6–12 g/day every 4–6 hrs.	Staphylococcal penicillin. Increase interval when creatinine clearance decreases. Hemorrhagic cystitis, platelet dysfunction, thrombocytopenia, nephropathy.
Metoclopramide (Reglan)	PO: 5 mg/5 mL syrup, 10 mg tabs. Parenteral: 5 mg/mL.	10–15 mg PO QID. Usually given 30 min before each meal and at bedtime.	Increases lower esophageal sphincter pressure and the rate of gastric emptying. Used as an antiemetic as well. Causes extrapyramidal symptoms and fatigue. Reduce dose and lengthen interval in renal failure.
Metolazone (Zaroxolyn)	PO: 2.5, 5, 10 mg tabs.	2.5–20 mg PO every day.	Has been useful when combined with a loop diuretic such as furosemide or ethacrynic acid. Side effects similar to those of thiazide diuretics.

TABLE 13–1. (cont.)
Common Drugs

Drug	How Supplied	Dose	Comments
Metoprolol (Lopressor)	PO: 50 and 100 mg tabs. IV: 5 mg/5 mL amps.	PO: 150–300 mg/day, usually given every 12 hrs.	Selective β-blocker.
Metronidazole (Flagyl)	PO: 250, 500 mg. Parenteral: 500 mg/100 mL NS.	IV: 7.5 mg/kg every 6–8 hrs. PO: 250–500 mg every 8 hrs.	Good anaerobic coverage. Used orally for trichomonas and *C. difficile* colitis.
Mexiletine (Mexitil)	150, 200, 250 mg capsules.	100–300 mg, PO every 6–8 hr.	Anti-arrhythmic. GI, CNS side effects. Can have arrhythmogenic effect.
Mezlocillin (Mezlin)	IM, IV diluted in 100 mg D5W or NS.	IM/IV: 18 g/day at dose of 3 g every 4 hrs.	Extended spectrum penicillin. Increase interval when creatinine clearance decreases. Thrombocytopenia, transient hyperbilirubinemia.
Mithramycin (Mithracin)	Vials of 2.5 mg/100 mg mannitol.	25 μg/kg body weight as single IV dose. May be given daily for 2–3 days or weekly over 3 wks.	Decreases serum calcium by a direct toxic effect on osteoclasts in bone. Very effective in hypercalcemia secondary to bone metastases. Causes anorexia, nausea, vomiting, thrombocytopenia, renal insufficiency, and hepatic dysfunction.

Nadolol (Corgard)	40, 80 mg tabs.	80–240 mg PO given once a day.	Nonselective β-blocker. Hydrophilic.
Nafcillin (Unipen, Natcil)	IM, IV diluted in 50–100 mL D5W or normal saline.	IV: 6–12 g/day every 6 hrs.	Anti-staphylococcal penicillin. No change for renal insufficiency. Platelet dysfunction, tissue damage with extravasation.
Naloxone hydrochloride (Narcan)	0.4 mg/mL in 1 mL container, 1 mg/mL in 2 mL container.	0.4–2.0 mg IV. May be repeated at 2–3-min intervals.	Narcotic antagonist. Adverse reactions include nausea, vomiting, diaphoresis, tachycardia, hypertension, and tremulousness. Note that once a desired effect has been obtained patients may need repeat administration to prevent a relapse of the narcotic effect.
Naproxen (Naprosyn)	250, 375, 500 mg tabs.	250–500 mg PO every 8 hrs not to exceed 1,250 mg/day.	Should not be used concomitantly with Anaprox since both circulate as the naproxen anion. Side effects similar to those of ibuprofen and indomethacin. Contraindicated in patients with the syndrome of nasal polyps, angioedema, and bronchospastic reactivity to aspirin.

TABLE 13–1. *(cont.)*
Common Drugs

Drug	How Supplied	Dose	Comments
Niacin (Nicobid, Nicolar)	50, 100 mg tabs. 125, 250 mg time-released tabs.	2-6 g/day given three to four times per day.	Flushing, pruritus, and gastrointestinal distress occur frequently. Therapy begun with small doses and advanced slowly. Patients receiving antihypertensive therapy may be at risk for postural hypotension.
Nifedipine (Procardia)	10, 20 mg capsules.	30–120 mg PO/day given every 6 to 8 hrs.	Calcium channel blocker. Works as potent vasodilator. Little effect on A-V nodal conduction.
Nitroglycerin (Nitrobid, Nitrostat)	Sublingual: 0.15, 0.3, 0.4, and 0.6 mg. Sustained release (oral): 2.5, 6.5, 9.0 mg. Ointment: 2.0%. Transdermal patch: 2.5, 5.0, 10, 15 mg. IV: diluted in 100 mg/250 mL D5W.	0.15–0.6 mg every 5–10 min. 2.5–9.0 mg every 8–12 hrs. 1–2 inches every 4–6 hrs. 2.5–15 mg/24 hrs. Start at 10–20 mcg per min and titrate.	Significant first pass hepatic metabolism with oral preparations. Tachyphylaxis with continuous use (oral and transdermal). Sublingual preparations should be replaced every 2 mo. Side effects are headache, postural hypotension, and reflex tachycardia.

Norepinephrine (Levophed)	4 mg amps diluted for IV infusion: 4 mcq/1 mL.	Begin with 16–24 mcg/min and titrate to desired effect.	α- and β-agonist. Preferential vasoconstriction in skin and skeletal muscle. Requires central line for administration.
Oxacillin (Prostaphlin)	IV, IM. Dilute in 50–100 mL NS or D5W.	IV/IM: 2–12 g/day every 4–6 hrs.	Anti-staphyloccal penicillin. No change for renal insufficiency. Transaminitis.
Paraldehyde	Parenteral: amps of 1 g/mL. PO: oral solution of 1 g/mL.	IV: diluted to 5% solution. 1.5–2.5 mL/kg by slow IV drip. IM: above dose by deep IM injection. May also be given rectally.	Anti-seizure medication. Produces sterile abscesses after IM injection. Dissolves plastic tubing. Contraindicated in hepatic or pulmonary disease. Should be used in status epilepticus after first line agents have failed.
Penicillin G	IM, IV, diluted in 50–100 mL D5W or NS.	IV/IM: 600,000–24 million U/day every 2–6 hrs.	1,600 U = 1 mg. Decrease higher doses for severe renal failure. May cause confusion and seizures.
Penicillin VK	PO: 250, 500 mg. Oral suspension: 250 mg/5 mL.	PO: 1–2 g/day every 6 hrs.	Lengthen interval when creatinine clearance decreases. Can cause confusion and seizures.

TABLE 13–1. (cont.)
Common Drugs

Drug	How Supplied	Dose	Comments
Pentamidine isoethion-ate (Pentam)	IM, IV. Diluted: 300 mg/ 100 mL for IV infusion with D5W or NS.	4 mg/kg/day IM or IV for 12–14 days. Usual dose 300 mg.	Alternative to trimethoprim-sulfame-thoxazole for pneumocystis. Side effects include: nephrotoxicity, hepatotoxicity, hypotension, neutropenia, and transient hypoglycemia.
Pentobarbital (Nembutal)	Parenteral: ampule, 100 mg/2 mL: vial, 2.5 g/50 mL. PO: 50 and 100 mg capsules.	IM: 150–200 mg. IV: 50 mg/min up to total of 200–500 mg. Should be given no faster than 50 mg/min. PO: 100 mg at bedtime as hypnotic. Rectal: 120–200 mg as hypnotic.	Parenteral form is only form useful as anticonvulsant. It is habit forming with chronic use. PO duration of action, 3–4 hrs. Dosage should be reduced in the elderly with impaired hepatic function, and with renal insufficiency. Side effects are somnolence, ataxia, confusion, hyperventilation, bradycardia, hypotension, and syncope.
Phenobarbital	Parenteral: 30 mg/mL, 60 mg/mL, 130 mg/mL vials. PO: 15, 30, 60, 100 mg tabs. 20 mg/5 mL elixir.	For status: 90–120 mg IV slow push, may be repeated every 10–15 min with 30–60 mg to a maximum dose of 500 mg. PO: 60–120 mg	Second line drug for status epilepticus. Respiratory depression common with IV therapy. Other side effects include drowsiness, hyperactivity, ataxia, skin eruptions, and megalo-blastic anemia. Serum concentra-

		tions of 15–40 mcg/mL recommended for control of seizures. It is a long acting barbiturate as opposed to pentobarbital, which is short-acting. Barbiturates contraindicated in acute intermittent porphyria.
	two to three times per day for chronic seizure disorder.	
Phenytoin (Dilantin)	Parenteral: 50mg/mL. PO: phenytoin sodium extended 100 mg capsules, phenytoin tabs 50 mg infatabs. Suspension: 125 mg/5 mL and 30 mg/5 mL.	IV loading dose: 1,000 mg at 50 mg/min; maintenance dose: 5 mg/kg/ day (300–400 mg every day may begin as single or divided doses IV or PO).	Anticonvulsant. IV administration at a rate faster than recommended may cause hypotension. IV preparation must be given slow IV push or diluted in saline. Side effects are GI upset, dermatitis, lupuslike syndrome, blood dyscrasias, gingival hypertrophy, and hirsutism. Phenytoin may also cause ataxia and nystagmus at toxic doses. Other side effects are megaloblastic anemia, lymphadenopathy, and liver damage. Drugs that increase phenytoin levels are isoniazid, coumadin, ethanol, ritalin, benzodiazepines, and phenothiazines. Therapeutic serum level 10–20 mcg/mL.

TABLE 13-1. *(cont.)*
Common Drugs

Drug	How Supplied	Dose	Comments
Piperacillin (Pipracil, others)	IM, IV diluted in 50–100 mL D5W or NS.	IM/IV: 12–24 g/day divided every 4 hrs.	Extended spectrum penicillin. Increase interval when creatinine clearance decreases. May cause platelet dysfunction and hypokalemia.
Potassium chloride (K-lyte Cl)	Available as powder in packets of 25 meq.	2.5 meq dissolved in 4–6 ounces of water two to four times per day as needed.	Dose depends on the needs of the patient. KCl is beneficial as a supplement to patients with hypokalemia and hypochloremic metabolic alkalosis. Common adverse reactions are nausea, vomiting, diarrhea, and abdominal pain.
(K-lor)	20 meq KCl/powder packet.		
(K-tab)	Tabs of 10 meq.		Extended release tab. Recommended for patients who cannot take liquid or effervescent potassium preparations.
Propylthiouracil	50 mg tabs. No parenteral form available.	Initial doses of 300–600 mg given three to four times a day are needed for control of symptoms. Usual maintenance	Mechanisms of action include inhibition of peripheral conversion of T4 to T3 and inhibition of tyrosine residues in thyroglobulin coupling. Higher doses necessary in thyroid storm. Side ef-

	dose is 100–300 mg in three divided doses.	fects include: granulocytopenia, pruritus, urticarial or papular rash, nausea, arthralgias, headache, dizziness, paresthesias, loss of taste, and drowsiness. Mild leukopenia may occur with doses greater than 400 mg/day.
Protamine sulfate	50 mg/5 mL container.	IV heparin <30 min: 1.5 mg/100 U heparin; 30–60 min: 0.75 mg/100 U heparin; >2 hrs: 0.375 mg/100 U heparin. SQ heparin: 1.0 mg/100 U heparin.	Indicated in heparin overdose. Contraindicated with a history of fish allergy or past intolerance. Protamine inactivates heparin catalytic activity. Hypotension occurs with rapid infusion, and over-dosage may cause hemorrhage.
Pseudoephedrine (Sudafed)	30 and 60 mg tabs. Liquid with 30 mg/5 mL.	30–60 mg PO QID.	Prescribed as a decongestant. Causes CNS stimulation. Hypertension or exacerbation of hypertension may occur.
Potassium phosphate	Powder concentrate 75 mL of solution supplies 250 mg phosphorus.	250 mg–2 g of phosphorus at meals and bedtime.	Must be dissolved in water. Neutraphos K contains 7.125 meq per 75 mL and neutraphos K contains 14.25 meq per 75 mL of reconstituted solution. May cause a laxative effect.

TABLE 13–1. (cont.)
Common Drugs

Drug	How Supplied	Dose	Comments
Prazosin (Minipress)	1, 2, and 5 mg capsules.	First dose should be 1 mg PO at bedtime.	Antihypertensive vasodilator. Causes first dose syncope and reflex tachycardia.
Probucol (Lorelco)	250 mg tabs.	500 mg PO BID.	Indicated for reduction of elevated serum cholesterol in patients with primary hypercholesterolemia. Associated with decreased HDL-cholesterol, but this has not been associated with decreased efficacy.
Procainamide (Pronestyl, others)	250, 375, 500 mg capsules, 100 mg/mL in 10 mL vial, 200 mg/mL in 2 mL amp. 250, 500 750 mg SR tabs.	PO load: 14 mg/kg. PO maintenance: 7 mg/kg every 4 hrs (every 6 hrs with SR prep). IM: 250–500 mg every 3–4 hrs. IV: load 100 mg every 5 hrs min to 1 g; maintenance: 1–4 mg/min.	Anti-arrhythmic. Prolongs QRS, QT, mental status changes, hypotension, rash, fever, 80% to 90% (+) ANA within 3–6 mos, 15% to 20% SLE syndrome. Should be discontinued if >50% prolongation of QRS during infusion. N-acetylprocainamide metabolite.
Propranolol (Inderal, Inderal LA)	Inderal: 10, 20, 40, 80 mg tabs. Inderal LA: 80, 120, 160 mg tabs.	120–400 mg/day given every 6–12 hrs. 120–400 mg once a day.	Nonselective β-blocker. Has high lipid solubility. Contraindicated in patients with CHF and bronchospasm. Angina may be precipitated with abrupt

discontinuation of β-blockers in patients at risk. Other side effects are hypotension, bradycardia, depression, fatigue, and rarely cytopenias. Use of β-blockers in diabetics may mask symptoms of hypoglycemia.

Pyridostigmine
(Mestinon)

Parenteral: 5 mg/mL. PO syrup: 60 mg/5 mL, tabs: 60 mg, timespan tabs: 180 mg.

Parenteral: 1/30th the oral dose IM or very slow IV. PO: 60–120 mg every 3–4 hrs. Intervals are shortened or lengthened as needed. Timespan tabs are dosed one to two times per day. Helpful for nightime use.

This drug is an anticholinesterase used in the treatment of myasthenia gravis. It increases the duration of action of acetylcholine released at the motor endplate. Doses may be increased before menstrual period or with infection. Ill patients refractory to the drug may improve with reduction or withdrawal of dose. Cholinergic crisis may be precipitated by overdosage, characterized by severe muscular weakness, dysphagia, and ventilatory failure. Edrophonium administraton with cholinergic crisis may produce deterioration. IV atropine is the treatment for cholinergic crisis. Other side effects are abdominal cramps, nausea, vomiting, diarrhea, salivation, diaphoresis, weakness, and muscle cramps. Contraindicated in patients with obstruction of the GI or urinary tract.

TABLE 13–1. (cont.)
Common Drugs

Drug	How Supplied	Dose	Comments
Quinidine (many brands)	200, 300 mg sulfate tabs. 324 mg gluconate tabs. Parenteral: 1 mL = 200 mg (sulfate) for IM use.	PO load: 12 mg/kg. Maintenance: 6 mg/kg every 4–6 hrs. Dose in terms of quinidine base.	Anti-arrhythmic. Prolongs QRS, QT, GI upset (decreased with gluconate), cinchonism, transaminitis, thrombocytopenia, proarrhythmic, fever, SLE syndrome.
Ranitidine (Zantac)	PO: 150 mg tablets. Parenteral: 25 mg/mL in 2 mL vials, diluted in 50 mL D5W.	150 mg PO BID or 300 mg PO at bedtime, 50 mg IV every 6–8 hrs.	H2 receptor antagonist. May cause malaise or dizziness. No antiandrogenic activity. Thrombocytopenia and granulocytopenia have been reported. Decrease dose in renal failure.
Rifampin	300 mg capsules.	600 mg PO every day.	Bactericidal to *Mycobacterium tuberculosis*. Also used for treatment of asymptomatic carriers of *Neisseria meningitidis*. Hepatotoxicity. Turns urine, sweat, tears red. Decreases effect of oral contraceptives, digoxin, steroids.
Spironolactone (Aldactone)	25 mg tabs.	25–50 mg PO BID to QID.	Is a potassium-sparing diuretic. Side effects include hyponatremia, hyper-

		kalemia, rash, and antiandrogen effects (gynecomastia, decreased libido, impotence, and galactorrhea).
Sodium nitroprusside (Nipride)	50 mg/5 mL amp diluted in 250 mL D5W.	0.5–10 mcg/kg/min IV.	Antihypertensive. Thiocyanate toxicity with prolonged use (more than 2-3 days), high doses, and renal insufficiency. Causes tinnitus, seizures, confusion, hyperreflexia, abdominal pain, and nausea.
Streptokinase (Streptase)	Powder dispensed to be reconstituted for IV use. Diluted up to 500 mL D5W or NS for IV infusion.	250,000 U load IV over 30 min followed by 100,000/hr for 24–72 hrs.	Indicated for acute massive pulmonary embolus, hemodynamically significant pulmonary embolus, extensive deep venous thrombosis, and acute myocardial infarction. Contraindications include recent cerebrovascular accident (within 2 mo), intracranial bleeding, recent surgery, and intracranial neoplasm. Past exposure to streptokinase is immunogenic. Side effects include allergic reactions, fever, hemorrhage, and phlebitis. Dosing not dependent on serum tests. Mechanism of action dependent on activating plasmin.

TABLE 13-1. (cont.)
Common Drugs

Drug	How Supplied	Dose	Comments
Sucralfate (Carafate)	1 g tabs.	1 g PO QID.	Poorly absorbed sulfated disaccharide forms an ulcer-adherent complex to enhance the mucosal barrier against gastric acid.
Sulfinpyrazone (Anturane)	200 mg capsules and 100 mg tabs.	100–200 mg PO BID initially. May be increased to 800 mg/day.	Not approved in United States as an antithrombotic agent. Used as a uricosuric agent.
Temazepam (Restoril)	15 mg, 30 mg capsules.	15–30 mg PO at bedtime.	Benzodiazepine hypnotic. t-1/2 of 15 hrs. Similar side effects as flurazepam.
Terbutaline (Brethine)	SQ: 2 mL ampuls with 1 mg/mL. PO: 2.5 and 5.0 mg tabs.	SQ: 0.25–0.35 mg every 20 min up to 0.5 mg total over 4 hrs or 1 mg over 24 hrs. PO: 2.5–5.0 mg every 4–6 hrs.	β-agonist bronchodilator. Onset and peak action similar to epinephrine (parenteral form). Side effects similar to epinephrine.
Terfenadine (Seldane)	60 mg tabs.	60 mg PO BID.	Pure H1 antagonist. Has minimal side effects but modest efficacy.
Tetracycline	PO: 250, 500 mg. Paren-	0.5–1 g every 12 hrs. IV:	Antibiotic. Fairly broad gram-positive

Drug	Preparation	Dose	Comments
	teral: diluted with at least 100 mL D5W or NS.	250–500 mg every 6 hrs PO.	and negative not *B. fragilis*. Covers chlamydia, rickettsia. Avoid in pregnancy and childhood due to enamel damage.
Theophylline (Theodur, Elixophyllin)	IV: theophylline for continuous infusion. PO: 100 mg, 200 mg, 300 mg tabs for theodur, a sustained release preparation. Concentration for IV infusion: 800 mg/500 mL. Oral liquid: 10 mg/mL.	IV: Bolus with 5–7.5 mg/kg over 30 min. Maintenance: smokers–0.6 mg/kg/hr; nonsmokers–0.4 mg/kg/hr; CHF, liver failure–0.2 mg/kg/hr. PO: take total IV dose over 24 hrs and give in divided doses. Oral liquid given every 6–8 hrs. Theodur given every 8–12 hrs. Theodur cannot be crushed; tab must be swallowed.	Methylxanthine bronchodilator. Theophylline is catabolized in the liver but excreted via the kidney. Clinically important drug interactions occur with erythromycin (decreases clearance), cimetidine and ranitidine (decrease clearance), phenytoin (increases clearance), and oral contraceptives (decrease clearance). t-1/2 is 4–5 hrs in smokers and 7–9 hrs in nonsmokers. Major toxicities include tachydysrhythmias, seizures, and GI upset. For serum levels >40 μg/mL induction of vomiting and the use of activated charcoal are indicated. Hemoperfusion is indicated for levels >60 μg/mL. Therapeutic levels 10–20 μg/mL.
Thiamine	Parenteral: 100 mg/mL. PO: 50 and 100 mg tabs.	100 mg PO, IM or IV recommended for early use in alcohol withdrawal.	Thiamine should be administered before glucose is administered in the alcoholic.

TABLE 13–1. (cont.)
Common Drugs

Drug	How Supplied	Dose	Comments
Ticarcillin (Ticar)	IM, IV diluted in 50–100 mL D5W or NS.	IM/IV: 200–300 mg/kg/day divided every 4 hrs.	Extended spectrum penicillin. Lengthen interval, decrease dose when creatinine clearance decreases. Hypernatremia/hypokalemia, platelet dysfunction. Can cause confusion, agitation.
Ticarcillin/clavulanic acid, (Timentin)	IV, IM: diluted in 100 mL NS or D5W.	3.1 g IV every 4 hrs.	Clavulanic acid broadens ticarcillin coverage to include β-lactamase organisms. Active against gram-positive (including staph), gram-negative (including *Hemophilus influenza*), anaerobes.
Tobramycin (Neocin)	IV, IM: diluted in 100 mL D5W or NS.	1.5 mg/kg every 8 hrs.	Aminoglycoside antibiotic. Active against aerobic gram-negative and staph. Nephrotoxic and ototoxic. Loading dose the same in renal disease but then must reduce and follow pre- and post-dose levels. Predose less than 2, 1 hour post-dose 4–10 desired.

Drug	Supplied	Dose	Notes
Tocainide (Tonocard)	400, 600 mg tabs.	200–800 mg every 8 hrs.	Anti-arrhythmic. Can cause shortened QT interval, GI upset, confusion, proarrhythmic, fever, agranulocytosis, hepatitis, and interstitial pneumonitis.
Triamterene (Dyrenium)	50 and 100 mg capsules.	50–100 mg PO BID.	Potassium-sparing diuretic. Similar to spironolactone. Dyazide is a preparation which contains triamterene and hydrochlorothiazide.
Triazolam (Halcion)	0.125 mg, 0.25, 0.5 mg tabs.	0.125–0.5 mg PO at bedtime.	Benzodiazepine hypnotic. Short t-1/2 of 2–3 hrs. Rebound insomnia after discontinuing the drug can occur.
Trihexyphenidyl HCL (Artane)	PO: 2 and 5 mg tabs, 2 mg/5 mL elixir.	1–15 mg in divided doses, usually TID. Usual starting dose is 1–2 mg.	Used as an anti-Parkinson agent and for extrapyramidal disorders. It inhibits the parasympathetic nervous system. May worsen glaucoma or urinary tract obstruction in patients with prostatic hypertrophy. Tardive dyskinesia may develop with long-term use. Side effects include dry mouth, dizziness, nausea, blurred vision, nervousness, and tachycardia.

TABLE 13–1. *(cont.)*
Common Drugs

Drug	How Supplied	Dose	Comments
Trimethoprim-sulfamethoxazole (Bactrim)	IV: 80 mg trimethoprim, 400 mg sulfamethoxasole per 5 mL. PO: 1 tab contains 80 mg trimethoprim and 400 mg sulfamethoxasole. Double-strength tab equivalent to 2 single strength tabs. Diluted in 125–500 mL D5W for IV use.	IV: usually 8–10 mg/kg (based on trimethoprim component) given in two to four divided doses. For pneumocystis, 15–20 mg/kg (based on trimethoprim component) given in three to four divided doses. PO: 1 double-strength tab every 12 hrs.	Antibiotic. Gram-positive, gram-negative, not enterococcus. Gram-negative, not *Pseudomonas aeruginosa.* Pneumocystis coverage at high dose. Rash, GI problems, thrombocytopenia, leukopenia.
Valproic acid (Depakane)	PO: 250 mg capsules, 250 mg/5 mL syrup.	Initial dose of 15 mg/kg/day. PO: increase by weekly intervals by 5–10 mg/kg/day. Usually given TID.	Contraindicated in patients with liver disease. This drug is hepatotoxic. Causes thrombocytopenia and platelet dysfunction. May cause false-positive results on urine ketones. May increase serum levels of phenobarbital and phenytoin. May also decrease serum phenytoin levels. Other side effects are nausea, vomiting, diarrhea, constipation, and abdominal cramps. May also cause pancreatitis.

Drug	Preparation	Dose	Comments
Vancomycin (Vancocin)	Oral capsules: 125 mg. Injection diluted in 100–250 mL D5W or NS.	IV: 1 g every 12 hrs. PO: 500 mg every 6 hrs.	Antibiotic. Gram-positive including methicillin-resistant staph, enterococcus. Oral form for *C. difficile* only. IV must give over 1 hr to avoid rash which often occurs if given too quickly. Can be nephrotoxic with aminoglycosides. Follow up levels: pre-dose less than 10, post-dose 20–40.
Vasopressin (Pitressin)	For parenteral use only: 20 U/mL.	0.5–1.5 U/min. Use IV infusion.	Vasoconstrictor. Has antidiuretic effect. May precipitate angina in susceptible patients. Causes tremor, diaphoresis, vertigo, circumoral pallor, abdominal cramping, vomiting, and urticaria.
Verapamil (Calan, Isoptin)	PO: 80 and 120 mg tabs, 240 mg SR tabs. IV: 5 mg/2 mL amps, 10 mg/4 mL amps.	240–480 every mg PO/day given every 8 hrs or 1 SR/day. 5–10 mg over 2–3 min. May repeat every third min prn.	Calcium channel blocker. Causes some vasodilatation. Has the greatest effect on A-V nodal conduction among the calcium channel blockers. Has negative inotropic effect.
Vitamin B12 (Cyanocobalamin)	Injection: 1 mL/100 mcg, 1 mL/1,000 mcg. Oral tabs: 100 mcg.	1,000 mcg IM every day for 1–2 wks. 1,000 mcg IM every wk for 4 wks or until Hct normalizes. 1,000 mcg IM every month for life.	Daily requirement: 2–5 μg. Response occurs within 48–72 hrs.

TABLE 13–1. *(cont.)*
Common Drugs

Drug	How Supplied	Dose	Comments
Vitamin K (Mephyton)	Tabs: 5 mg. Parenteral: 1 mL = 10 mg.	2.5–10 mg SQ or IM. IV not recommended.	Indicated for hypothrombinemia secondary to anticoagulant use, malabsorption, or dietary insufficiency. May require repeat dose if prothrombin does not normalize.
Warfarin (Coumadin)	2, 2.5, 5, 7.5, and 10 mg tabs.	10 mg PO initially and then 4–16 mg PO every day. Adjust protime to 1.5–2.0 times the control or 15% to 35% activity.	Indicated as prophylaxis for recurrent thromboembolic disease and atrial fibrillation with embolization. Contraindications similar to heparin. Also contraindicated in pregnancy. Prevents complete synthesis of vitamin K dependent factors (II, VII, IX, X). Complications include hemorrhage and dermatitis. Potentiation of effect caused by concurrent use of anabolic steroids, cimetidine, metronidazole, thrombolytics, thyroid supplements, clofibrate, salicylates, and quinidine. Effect is inhibited by ethanol, barbiturates, corticosteroids, estrogens, carbamazepine, and rifampin.

Anti-Emetics		
Prochlorperazine (Compazine)	5, 10 mg tabs. Spansule capsules 10, 15, and 30 mg. 2 mL ampules at 5 mg/mL. Multidose vials of 10 mL at 5 mg/mL, syrup 5 mg/5 mL, suppositories 25 mg.	5–10 mg three to four times a day, 10 mg capsule every 12 hrs, 5–10 mg IM every 3–4 hrs, not to exceed 40 mg/day. Suppositories: 25 mg BID.	Adverse reactions are dystonias, extrapyramidal effects, motor restlessness, drowsiness, dizziness, leukopenia, cholestasis.
Trimethobenzamide (Tigan)	100 and 250 mg capsules, 200 mg suppositories, 100 mg/mL in 2 and 20 mL containers.	250 mg TID caps, 200 mg TID suppositories, 200 mg TID IM: IV dose not recommended.	Same as above.
Metoclopramide (Reglan)	IV form only 5 mg/mL in 2, 10, 30 mL containers.	10 mg IV before chemotherapy.	Used for prevention of nausea and vomiting with chemotheapy.
Promethazine (Phenergan)	12.5, 25, 50 mg tabs, 12.5, 25, 50 mg suppositories.	25 mg PO or rectally every 4–6 hrs.	Less antidopaminergic effects. Less effective in vomiting due to toxins or radiation. More effective in prevention of motion sickness.

TABLE 13-2.
Oral Corticosteroids Comparison Chart*

Duration and Drug	Equivalent Anti-inflammatory Dose (mg)	Relative Anti-inflammatory Potency	Relative Mineralo-corticoid Activity	Dosage-Forms	Plasma Half-life (Hrs)	Comments
Triamcinolone	4	5	0	Tab 1, 2, 4, 8, 16 mg Syrup 400, 800 mcg/ml	3.3+	May cause a higher frequency of muscle wasting
Long-acting (biologic activity 36-54 hr)						
Betamethasone	0.6	25	0	Tab 600 mcg Syrup 120 mcg/ml	—	Minimal sodium re-taining activity, but with high doses retention may occur.
Dexamethasone	0.75	30	0	Tab 250, 500, 750 mcg 1.5, 4 mg Elxr 100 mcg/ml	Men 3.4 Women 2.4	
Mineralocorticoid (biologic activity 12-24 hr)						
Fluorocortisone	—	10	125	Tab 100 mcg	—	Mineralocorticoid useful in Addison's disease.

Short-Acting (biologic activity less than 12 hr)						
Cortisone	25	0.8	0.8	Tab 5, 10, 25 mg	0.5	Must be hydroxylated to active species (hydrocortisone)
Hydrocortisone	20	1	1	Tab 5, 10, 20 mg / Susp 2 mg/ml	1.5	Daily secretion in man = 20 mg
Intermediate-Acting (biologic activity) 12–36 hr						
Prednisone	5	4	0.8	Tab 1, 2.5, 5, 10, 20, 50 mg	3.6	Must be hydroxylated to active species (prednisone)
Prednisolone	5	4	0.8	Tab 1, 2.5, 5 mg	3	Minimal sodium-retaining activity
Methylprednisolone	4	5	0.5	Tab 2, 4, 8, 16, 24, 32 mg	3.3	Minimal sodium-retaining activity

*From Knoben JE, Pharm D, Anderson PO, et al (eds): *Handbook of Clinical Drug Data*, ed 6. Hamilton, Il, Drug Intelligence Publications, Inc, 1988, pp 667–668. Used by permission.

TABLE 13–3.
Insulin*

Type	Preparation	Time of Onset (Hr)	Duration of Action (Hr)	Peak Effect (Hr)
Short-acting	Regular insulin	1	6–8	2–4
	Semilente insulin	1	10–14	2–6
Intermediate-acting	NPH insulin	2	18–24	6–12
	Lente insulin	2	18–24	6–12
Long-acting	Protamine zinc insulin	7	36	14–24
	Ultralente insulin	7	36	18–24

*Insulin is available as beef, pork, mixture of beef and pork, and human insulin.

TABLE 13-4.
Laxatives

Drug	How Supplied	Onset of Action	Dose	Comments
Psyllium hydrophilic colloid (Metamucil)	As powder.	12–72 hrs.	1 tsp PO one to three times a day.	Bulk forming agent to be taken with water. Danger of impaction or obstruction if narrowing present in alimentary canal. May cause allergic reactions.
Bisacodyl (Dulcolax)	5 mg or 10 mg tabs.	6–12 hrs.	2–3 tabs PO every day or 1 suppository every day.	Stimulant. Tablets must be swallowed whole. Dissolution in stomach causes dyspepsia. Do not take with antacids or milk. Can cause diarrhea and hypokalemia. This class of laxatives is most frequently abused. Do not use for more than 1 wk on a continuous basis. In severe abuse, can stimulate megacolon.
Docusate sodium (Colace)	50 and 100 mg capsules, liquid 10 mg/mL, syrup 20 mg/5 mL.	1–3 days.	50–200 mg a day in one to two doses.	Wetting agent used for constipation produced by delay in rectal emptying.

TABLE 13-4. (cont.)
Laxatives

Drug	How Supplied	Onset of Action	Dose	Comments
Casanthranol and docusate sodium (Peri-colace)	Capsules containing 30 mg casanthranol and 100 mg docusate sodium.	8–12 hrs.	1–2 capsules a day in one to two doses.	Combination of mild stimulant laxative and stool softener.
Mineral Oil	As an emulsion.	...	15–45 mL PO BID.	Prolonged use causes fat malabsorption. Should not be used with a wetting agent because of increased absorption and hepatic infiltration. Causes pruritis ani. Acts as foreign agent in a wound. Aspiration causes lipoid pneumonia.
Magnesium citrate	Present in solution as 1.5–1.9 g/dL magnesium oxide with citric acid and potassium bicarbonate.	2–6 hrs.	200 mL PO.	Saline cathartic useful in eliminating parasites. Used to decrease transit time with poison ingestion. Contraindicated in renal failure.

TABLE 13–5.
Pain Medications

Drug	How Supplied	Dose	Comments
Morphine sulfate	Parenteral solution as 2, 4, 10, 15 mg/mL; or 10, 15, 30 mg tabs.	IM, SQ: 5–20 mg; IV: 2.5–15 mg. May also be used as continuous IV infusion.	Adverse reactions are respiratory depression, nausea, vomiting, hypotension, bradycardia, increased intracranial pressure, constipation, histamine release, spasm of biliary tract, urinary retention, miosis, and hypersensitivity reactions. The oral form is less active.
MS Contin (morphine sulfate in controlled-release form)	30 mg tabs.	Given every 12 hrs PO.	Used for chronic pain. Use 1:3 ratio for parenteral:oral conversion.
Hydromorphone hydrochloride (Dilaudid)	2 mg/mL in 1 mL containers; 2, 3, 4 mg/mL in 2 mL containers.	1–2 mg every 4–6 hrs IM, SQ; 1–2 mg every 4 hrs slow IV push.	Adverse effects same as above.
Meperidine hydrochloride (Demerol)	Multiple containers and concentrations.	IM, IV, SQ 100 mg every 3–4 hrs.	Adverse effects same as above. Dose decreased in liver failure. Contraindicated in renal failure because of the accumulation of pharmacologically active metabolites.
Levorphanol tartrate (Levo-Dromoran formulation)	2 mg tabs, 2 mg/mL in 1 mL and 10 mL containers.	2–3 mg every 4–6 hrs.	Four to eight times as potent as morphine. Longer acting and more effective than morphine given orally.

TABLE 13–5. *(cont.)*
Pain Medications

Drug	How Supplied	Dose	Comments
Butorphanol tartrate (Stadol)	1 mg/mL in 1 mL containers; 2 mg/mL in 1, 2, 10 mL containers.	IM: 2 mg every 3–4 hrs. IV: 1–2 mg every 3–4 hrs.	Do not give to patients dependent on opiates because of antagonist properties.
Methadone hydrochloride (Dolophine Hydrochloride)	10 mg/mL in 1 and 20 mL containers; 5 and 10 mg tabs.	2.5–10 mg SQ or IM every 3–4 hrs, 2.5–10 mg PO every 6 hrs.	Drug interaction with rifampin necessitates increase in the dose of methadone.
Codeine with acetaminophen (Tylenol no. 3)	Each tab contains 300 mg acetaminophen and 30 mg codeine phosphate. Elixir 12 mg codeine/5 mL teaspoon.	1–2 tabs PO every 4–6 hrs. 15 mL PO every 4 hrs.	Adverse effects: drowsiness, constipation, respiratory depression, nausea, and emesis. Overdose may cause hepatic necrosis.

TABLE 13–6.
Sulfonylureas

Drug	How Supplied	Dose	Comments
Acetohexamide (Dymelor)	250 mg and 500 mg.	250–1,500 mg in one or two doses.	Duration of action 12–18 hrs. Hypoglycemia, cholestatic jaundice, allergic reactions, and leukopenia are side effects.
Tolbutamide (Orinase)	250 mg and 500 mg.	250 mg–3.0 g divided into two to three doses.	Duration of action 6–12 hrs.
Chlorpropamide (Diabenese)	100 mg and 250 mg.	100 mg–500 mg once a day.	Long duration of action: 36–60 hrs. Watch for prolonged hypoglycemia. Can cause hyponatremia similar to SIADH effect. Highly protein bound. May potentiate hypoglycemic effect when administered with other highly protein bound drugs.
Glipizide (Glucotrol)	5 mg and 10 mg.	2.5–40 mg; doses > 15 mg should be given BID.	Duration of action is 12–24 hrs.
Glyburide (DiaBeta and Micronase)	1.25, 2.5, and 5.0 mg.	1.25–20 mg.	Duration of action is 18–24 hrs. Second generation sulfonylureas have been given in addition to insulin.

Procedures

Richard Petrak, M.D.
Stephen Paul, M.D.

ARTERIAL BLOOD GAS

A. Radial artery puncture.
1. Place patient's arm on a flat surface.
2. Extend wrist 30° to 45°.
3. Palpate artery 1–2 cm proximal to the distal end of the radius at the wrist.
4. Clean area with an alcohol swab.
5. Coat the walls of a 3-mL syringe with heparin, or use a previously heparinized syringe.
6. Attach syringe to a 23G butterfly needle.
7. Hold the needle by the butterfly and palpate the artery with your other hand.
8. Pointing the needle proximally, enter the skin over the artery at an angle somewhere between 45° and 90° (Fig 14–1).
9. Advance needle slowly. Once in the artery, blood should pulsate in the butterfly tubing.
10. Collect 1–2 mL of blood.
11. Withdraw needle and apply firm pressure to the puncture wound for 5 minutes.
12. Meanwhile, hold syringe vertically with needle upward and expel air bubbles from the sample.
13. Cap the syringe tightly and place it in ice.
14. Have sample analyzed immediately.

B. Femoral artery puncture.
1. Have the patient lie supine with leg mildly abducted and externally rotated.

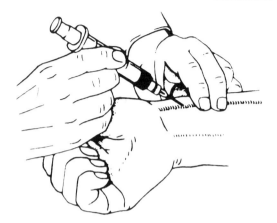

FIG 14–1
Collection of an arterial sample. (From Suratt, Gibson (eds): *Manual of Medical Procedures.* St Louis, CV Mosby Co, 1982. Used by permission.)

    2. Locate the artery 2 cm distal to the inguinal ligament (Fig 14–2).
    3. With a heparinized syringe and a 22G straight needle, enter skin overlying the artery at a 90° angle.
    4. Aspirate while advancing toward the artery.
    5. Once in the artery, collect 1–2 mL of blood.
    6. Remove needle, apply pressure for 5 minutes, evacuate the bubbles from the syringe, and place specimen on ice.
  C. Brachial artery puncture.
    1. Position patient's arm fully extended at the elbow.
    2. Locate the artery medial to the biceps brachii tendon and at the level of the antecubital fossa (Fig 14–3).

3. Use technique as described previously for radial artery puncture.

BLOOD CULTURES

A. Rub area vigorously with alcohol.
B. Apply iodine/povidine solution to area.
C. Do not touch sterile area with anything except other sterile objects.
D. Sterilize rubber diaphragm of each blood culture bottle.
E. Draw 10 mL of blood from sterile area with a sterile needle.

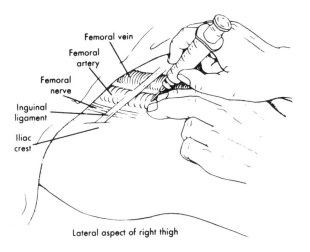

Femoral vein
Femoral artery
Femoral nerve
Inguinal ligament
Iliac crest

Lateral aspect of right thigh

FIG 14–2
Technique of femoral artery puncture. First two fingers of free hand are used to palpate femoral artery. (From Suratt, Gibson (eds): *Manual of Medical Procedures*. St Louis, CV Mosby Co, 1982. Used by permission.)

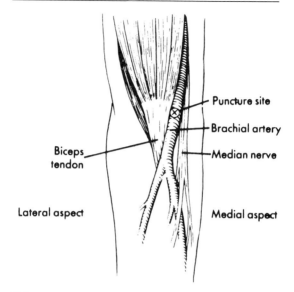

FIG 14–3
Anatomic site for brachial artery puncture. Approximate point of entry into vessel is indicated with *X*. (From Suratt, Gibson (eds): *Manual of Medical Procedures.* St Louis, CV Mosby Co, 1982. Used by permission.)

    F. Replace the first needle with another sterile needle.
    G. Place 5 mL of blood in one culture bottle.
    H. Replace the second needle with a third sterile needle.
    I. Place 5 mL of blood into another culture bottle.

THORACENTESIS
    A. Have the patient sit upright with arms resting on a table in front of him.

B. Percuss the posterior thorax from superior to inferior and locate the superior margin of dullness.

C. Mark a spot for thoracentesis (i.e., posterolateral chest about one to two interspaces below the superior margin of dullness and in the most inferior aspect of the interspace; see Fig 14–4).

D. Disinfect area and drape under sterile conditions.

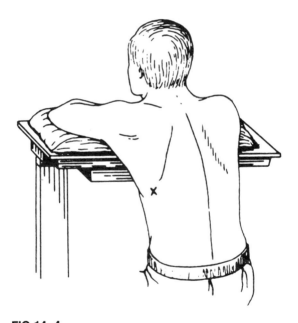

FIG 14–4

Patient position. (From Suratt, Gibson (eds): *Manual of Medical Procedures*. St Louis, CV Mosby Co, 1982. Used by permission.)

E. Anesthetize area superficially with 1% lidocaine using a 25G needle, then switch to a 20G needle.

F. Enter the skin with a 20G needle in the anesthetized area. Needle and syringe should be held at a 90° angle to the skin.

G. Aspirate while advancing slowly.

H. If you hit the rib, inject a small amount of lidocaine and "walk" the needle over the rib, continue to advance slowly while aspirating.

I. Stop once in the pleural space (noted by pleural fluid entering syringe). At this juncture, one can unscrew the syringe from the needle, and place another sterile syringe on the needle to aspirate the desired quantity of fluid. Alternately, one could use a thoracentesis kit. Aspirate no more than 1 L of pleural fluid.

J. Order a chest x-ray after the procedure to rule out pneumothorax.

THORACENTESIS KIT DIRECTIONS

A. Once the area is anesthetized with lidocaine and the pleural space is entered, withdraw the needle and syringe while applying pressure to the puncture site with sterile gauze.

B. Take a large-bore needle, a 60-mL syringe, one-way valve, tubing, and a specimen bag from the kit.

C. Attach as shown in the diagram in the kit.

D. Insert the needle as done previously in the anesthetized area. Advance slowly while applying negative pressure to the syringe.

E. Once fluid enters the syringe, advance no further.

F. Move the needle guard down to the skin and lock it there to prevent any further advancement of the needle.

G. Aspirate until the syringe is full. Positive pressure on the plunger of the syringe will force fluid through the valve into the specimen bag.

H. Do not aspirate more than 1 L of fluid.

FOLEY CATHETER

A. Men.
1. Patient should be supine with legs slightly apart.
2. Saturate gauze with antiseptic solutions.
3. Put on sterile gloves.
4. Thoroughly wash penis with antiseptic solution.
5. Lubricate catheter down the length of the tube.
6. Hold penis and stretch at right angle to the body.
7. Insert lubricated catheter slowly through the urethral meatus (Fig 14–5).
8. Advance catheter as far as the hub of the balloon inflation tip.
9. Inject 5 mL saline via inflation tip.
10. Pull catheter back until some resistance is met.
11. Tape catheter to one thigh with a short piece of tape.

B. Women.
1. Patient should be supine with legs widely spread.
2. Spread labia until the urethral meatus is visualized.
3. Sterilize area.
4. Lubricate catheter, advance slowly and inflate balloon once urine returns.
5. Tape catheter to one thigh.

GRAM STAIN

A. Apply specimen to glass slide so that only a thin layer remains.
B. Allow specimen to air dry.
C. Heat fix specimen by placing the opposite side of the slide over the flame until the slide is warm to touch (takes only seconds to accomplish this).
D. Flood the slide with crystal violet solution, let stand for a few seconds, and rinse under tap water.
E. Flood the slide with Gram's iodine, allow to stand for a few seconds, and rinse.

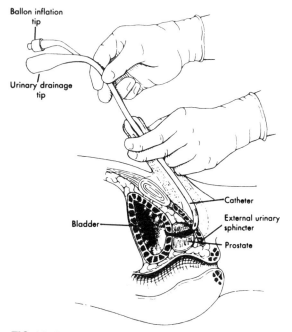

FIG 14–5
Passing the catheter. (From Suratt, Gibson (eds): *Manual of Medical Procedures*. St Louis, CV Mosby Co, 1982. Used by permission.)

F. Hold the slide at a slight angle, apply decolorizer and allow decolorizer to run off slide immediately. Apply decolorizer until the slide loses its purple tinge, then rinse with water.

G. Flood slide with safranin, allow to stand for a few seconds, and rinse.

H. Dry slide with tissue.

VENOUS BLOOD DRAW (FEMORAL)

A. Have patient lie flat in bed with leg slightly abducted and externally rotated.
B. Palpate femoral artery 2 cm inferior to the inguinal
   ligament. (The femoral vein is just medial to the artery at this level.)
C. Sterilize area.
D. Select search needle.
E. With fingertips on the femoral artery, enter the skin
   medially at a 90° angle to the plane of the skin.
F. Aspirate once under the skin and advance the needle
   slowly until blood is returned.

LUMBAR PUNCTURE

A. Bed should be flat.
B. Place patient in the lateral decubitus fetal position
   (i.e., knees up to chest and head bent as far forward
   as possible). The patient's back should be as close
   to the edge of the bed as possible.
C. Fully expose lumbar sacral spines (Fig 14–6).
D. Sterilize lumbar sacral area with povidone-iodine solution and sponges supplied in the kit.
E. Drape area so that only area in question is exposed.
   The puncture should be done between L4 and L5
   vertebrae. To find this space, palpate the superior iliac crest; L4–5 is directly medial to that point.
F. Anesthetize superficially with a 25G needle.
G. Change needle to 21G to anesthetize deeper. Advance needle by palpating the superior edge of L5
   and placing the needle slightly superior to that.
   Needle should be pointed toward the umbilicus and
   held at a 90° angle to the patient (or parallel to the
   bed). Advance needle slowly, aspirating along the
   way. If resistance is not met inject lidocaine, redirect needle, and proceed. Once the needle can go no
   further, pull back slowly and inject lidocaine along
   the tract.
H. Take a 21G spinal needle and check that the stylet
   can be easily removed and replaced. Enter the skin

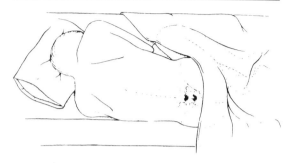

FIG 14–6
Lateral decubitus position. (From Suratt, Gibson (eds): *Manual of Medical Procedures*. St Louis, CV Mosby Co, 1982. Used by permission.)

with the bevel up. It is helpful to hold the spinal needle between the thumbs at the most distal end and between the tips of the forefingers at the proximal end. This helps to steady the needle while advancing. Advance the needle slowly in the same manner as discussed in step G (Fig 14–7).

I. If resistance is met, stop, pull the needle back, redirect the needle tip, and advance again.

J. One may feel a decrease in resistance (often referred to as a "pop") on passing through the arachnoid layer and into the subarachnoid space. At that point, turn the needle 90° so that the bevel faces cephalad. If in the subarachnoid space, cerebrospinal fluid should come through the needle promptly on removal of the stylet.

K. If unable to obtain fluid in the lateral decubitus position, it may be easier to position the patient seated as in Fig 14–4. Enter the skin in the same location, but direct the needle 30° down from parallel.

L. Attach a manometer to the hub of the needle to measure the opening pressure.

    M. Collect specimens. When done, insert stylet once
       again, turn needle 90° so the bevel is up, and re-
       move the needle slowly.

    N. Puncture site should require only a minimal amount
       of pressure to stop bleeding and an adhesive band-
       age should suffice for covering this site.

ABDOMINAL PARACENTESIS

    A. Place the patient in a supine position. Make certain
       the patient's bladder is empty.

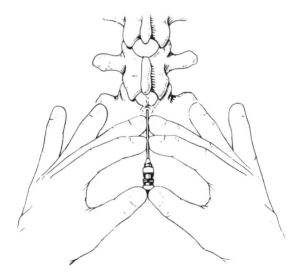

FIG 14–7
Insert spinal needle into subcutaneous tissue and advance
needle into subarachnoid space. (From Suratt, Gibson (eds):
Manual of Medical Procedures. St Louis, CV Mosby Co,
1982. Used by permission.)

    B. Select one of the following puncture sites:
        1. Point in midline, midway between the symphysis pubis and umbilicus (location of choice for patients with a coagulopathy).
        2. Point in either lower abdominal flank lateral to the rectus muscle.
    C. Sterilize the area and wear sterile gloves.
    D. Anesthetize the skin and then deep tissues down to and including the peritoneum.
    E. Hold an 18G intracatheter needle at a 90° angle to the skin and advance slowly. Entry through the peritoneum will be indicated by a pop or a give.
    F. Withdraw the needle, leaving the catheter in the abdomen.
    G. Attach a 20-mL syringe and aspirate to collect fluid.
    H. Remove catheter and apply sterile absorbent dressing.

ENDOTRACHEAL INTUBATION

    A. Oral tracheal tube insertion.
        1. Clear airway of secretions, vomitus, dentures, etc.
        2. Ventilate the patient with 100% oxygen with a bag and mask if the patient is hypoxic, apneic, or hypercarbic.
        3. Select the endotracheal tube (ETT) and inflate balloon, checking for leaks.
        4. Deflate and lubricate the distal end, including the cuff.
        5. Anesthetize the pharynx and larynx if the patient is awake.
        6. Position patient's head on a 10 cm (4 inch) pillow or pad in a slightly extended position.
        7. Open mouth by extending the jaw with your right hand. Hold laryngoscope in your left hand and insert blade in the right side of the mouth so that it pushes the tongue to the left. Advance blade until the epiglottis appears. If using a curved blade, place it in the vallecula (space

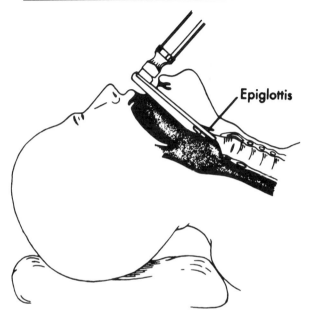

FIG 14-8
Placement of tip of straight laryngoscope. (From Suratt, Gibson (eds): *Manual of Medical Procedures*. St Louis, CV Mosby Co, 1982. Used by permission.)

between the epiglottis and the base of the tongue). When using a straight blade, place it just beyond the epiglottis (Fig 14-8).

8. Expose the larynx by lifting the laryngoscope handle with your left arm and shoulder upward and forward. Hold your wrist rigid and do not rotate the tip of the blade while using the teeth

as a fulcrum. If larynx cannot be readily seen, have an assistant put slight pressure on the thyroid cartilage.

9. Place the ETT into the trachea by holding it in your right hand with bevel up and toward the right. Insert tube into the mouth and slide it along the right side into the trachea until the cuff just disappears past the vocal cords. If the tube cannot be inserted because it flexes in the wrong direction, remove the tube and insert a stylet in it. Bend the ETT and stylet in proper curvature to conform with the patient's pharynx (hockey stick conformation).

10. Once past the vocal cords with the cuff, pull out the stylet (if used), attach a ventilation bag immediately, and resume ventilation.

11. Inflate the cuff with 10 mL of air or with enough air to prevent a leak around the cuff.

12. Auscultate the chest, checking for breath sounds bilaterally. Breath sounds more prominent on the right than left suggests that the right mainstem bronchus has been intubated. In this case, deflate the cuff, pull the ETT back a few centimeters, inflate the cuff, and auscultate again.

13. Tape the ETT securely in place to prevent it from sliding out of the trachea or down the right mainstem bronchus.

14. Obtain a chest x-ray to confirm placement of the ETT.

HEIMLICH TUBE INSERTION

A. Place the patient in a supine position.

B. Sterilize the area of the seventh intercostal space in the anterior axillary line on the side of the pneumothorax.

C. Take a Heimlich tube and remove the cap from the needle.

D. Insert the needle at a 90° angle to the skin in the

seventh intercostal space just superior to the eighth rib and advance gradually. On entry into the pleural space, a gush of air should come through the one-way valve.

E. Alternatively, if a Heimlich tube is unavailable, attach an 18G needle to the intravenous (IV) tubing. Insert the distal end of the IV tubing into a container of water to ensure a water seal. Insert the needle as in step D.

F. Secure the tube in place.

G. Plan for chest tube insertion.

CENTRAL LINES

A. General principles.

1. Assess the patient for distorted anatomy (Fig 14–9).

2. Make sure coagulation studies and the platelet count are adequate.

3. Determine if the patient can tolerate Trendelenburg.

4. Explain the procedure and complications to the patient.

5. Assemble equipment: catheter set with 14G or 16G 6-cm needle and a guidewire, prep and draping material, 1% lidocaine (10 mL), heparin flushes (if using triple lumen set), 25G and 22G needles, two syringes (5 or 10 cm), and suture (3-0 silk on a straight needle).

6. Position patient and find landmarks.

7. Prepare area and drape.

8. Anesthetize the skin with lidocaine.

9. A "search" needle (22G needle on syringe) is first used to cannulate the vein. This is especially useful for inexperienced people to decrease the complication rate.

10. Always maintain negative pressure whether inserting the needle or removing it (if bright red blood flows rapidly into the syringe, the carotid artery has been cannulated. Immediately re-

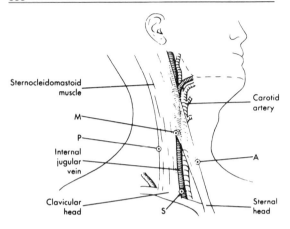

FIG 14–9

Anatomic landmarks. Common approaches to venipuncture are anterior (*A*), medial (*M*), posterior (*P*), and suprasternal (*S*). (From Suratt, Gibson (eds): *Manual of Medical Procedures.* St Louis, CV Mosby Co, 1982. Used by permission.)

          move the needle and apply ample pressure to the artery for 5 to 10 minutes).

11. If there is no blood flow after proper insertion of the needle, withdraw the needle slowly while maintaining negative pressure as you may enter the lumen on withdrawal of the needle.

12. If there is no blood return, remove the needle and reassess landmarks and the patient's position and reinsert the needle at a different angle.

B. Internal jugular vein.

There are 4 approaches, 3 of which will be discussed in this text. The fourth is the anterior approach, which is falling out of favor because of a high complication rate.

   1. Central approach.

      a. Position the patient in Trendelenburg at 15°,

with head turned to the opposite side. The right side is the preferred site of entry.

b. Define landmarks: locate the triangle formed by the sternal and clavicular heads of the sternocleidomastoid muscle and the clavicle. The internal jugular vein runs through this triangle before it enters the subclavian vein.

c. Locate the carotid artery and, if possible, palpate and retract it medially.

d. Insert the search needle at the apex of the triangle (Fig 14–10).

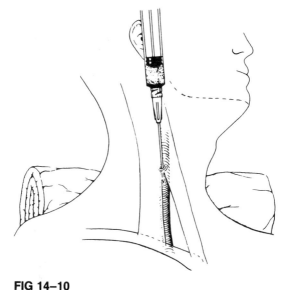

FIG 14–10
Insert "seeking" needle. Aim for ipsilateral nipple and aspirate. (From Suratt, Gibson (eds): *Manual of Medical Procedures*. St Louis, CV Mosby Co, 1982. Used by permission.)

e. Direct the needle caudally and laterally at a 45° angle aiming toward the ipsilateral nipple (remember to maintain negative pressure).

f. If unsuccessful, direct needle 5° to 10° laterally and try again. Do not go medially as the carotid artery is located there.

g. Once the vein is entered, pull the search needle out maintaining landmarks, and introduce a larger needle in the same manner.

h. Once the vein is entered with the large needle, take the syringe off and place your thumb over the distal end of the needle to prevent air from entering the vein. The catheter is introduced either directly or over the guide wire. If entering the catheter directly through the needle, pass it slowly, being cautious not to pull the catheter back, as the needle could shear the catheter, causing part of the catheter to embolize.

i. If using a guide wire, *never* let go of the wire.

j. Secure catheter to the skin with 3-0 silk sutures.

2. Posterior approach.

a. Position the patient in Trendelenburg at 15° with head turned to opposite side.

b. Define landmarks: locate the external jugular vein, lateral border of the sternocleidomastoid muscle, clavicle, and the suprasternal notch.

c. Insert the search needle at the lateral border of the sternocleidomastoid muscle just posterior to the junction of the external jugular vein and the posterior edge of the clavicular head of the sternocleidomastoid muscle. If you cannot locate the external jugular vein, enter the skin between the middle and lower third of the sternocleidomastoid muscle at the lateral border (Fig 14–11).

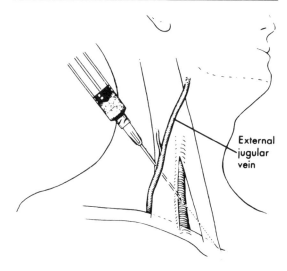

FIG 14–11
Insert "seeking" needle. Aim for suprasternal notch and aspirate. (From Suratt, Gibson (eds): *Manual of Medical Procedures*. St Louis, CV Mosby Co, 1982. Used by permission.

> d. Aim the search needle caudally and ven-
>   trally toward the suprasternal notch at a 45°
>   angle maintaining a plane just posterior to
>   the sternocleidomastoid muscle.
> e. The vein should be entered at 5–7 cm.
> f. If unsuccessful, assess landmarks and try
>   again.
> g. Once the vein is cannulated, follow steps H
>   to J of the central approach.
> 3. Subclavian approach.
>   a. Position: place the patient at a 15° Trende-
>   lenburg to distend the subclavian vein.

Place a rolled sheet between the patient's scapulae to better define the desired landmarks. Turn the patient's head to the opposite side.

b. Define landmarks: locate the suprasternal notch, and a point between the middle and lateral third of the clavicle (the most depressed part of clavicle).

c. Insert a search needle parallel to the anterior chest wall 1–2 cm caudal to the clavicle directing the needle just beneath the clavicle aiming at the suprasternal notch (Fig 14–12).

d. Advance the needle, keeping it parallel to the chest wall and as close to the caudal

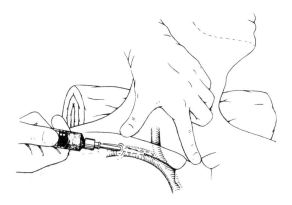

FIG 14–12
Insert cannulation needle. Aim for suprasternal notch. Advance needle as close to underside of clavicle as possible and aspirate. (From Suratt, Gibson (eds): *Manual of Medical Procedures.* St Louis, CV Mosby Co, 1982. Used by permission.)

edge of the clavicle as possible.

    e. Once the vein is entered, withdraw the search needle maintaining landmarks and introduce a larger needle in similar fashion.

    f. Once the large needle is in the vein, rotate the needle caudally 90° to facilitate a downward direction of the catheter tip.

    g. Now follow steps H to J of the central approach.

C. Femoral vein.

    1. Position: patient is flat in bed with leg extended slightly, abducted and externally rotated (Fig 14–2).

    2. Landmarks: locate the femoral artery either with pulsation or by finding the midpoint of a line drawn between the anterior iliac spine and the symphysis pubis.

    3. Insert a large needle medial to the artery at a 45° angle to the frontal plane and two fingerbreaths below the inguinal ligament.

    4. If unsuccessful, pull the needle out and assess landmarks. Then re-insert the needle more medially.

    5. Once the vein is entered, follow steps H to J of the central approach.

BIBLIOGRAPHY

Surrah, Gibson (eds): *Manual of Medical Procedures*. St. Louis, CV Mosby Co, 1982.

Index

T